P ED 28 $9.95 K1

D11195289

WON'T YOU JOIN THE DANCE?

"What matters it how far we go?" his scaly friend
      replied.
"There is another shore, you know, upon the other
      side.
The further off from England the nearer is to
      France—
Then turn not pale, beloved snail, but come and
      join the dance.
    Will you, won't you, will you, won't you, will
      you join the dance?
    Will you, won't you, will you, won't you, won't
      you join the dance?"

      —From the Lobster Quadrille in
      Lewis Carroll's *Alice's Adventures in Wonderland*

# WON'T YOU JOIN

MAYFIELD PUBLISHING COMPANY

# THE DANCE?

## A Dancer's Essay into the Treatment of Psychosis

TRUDI SCHOOP
with Peggy Mitchell

Illustrations by Hedi Schoop

Copyright © 1974 by Trudi Schoop and Peggy Mitchell

First edition 1974

All rights reserved. No portion of this book may
be reproduced in any form or by any means
without written permission of the publisher.

Library of Congress Catalog Card Number: 73-87475
International Standard Book Numbers: 0-87484-229-8

Manufactured in the United States of America

Supervising editor was Richard W. Bare and production
editor was Liselotte Hofmann. Michelle Hogan
supervised production, and designer was Nancy Sears.

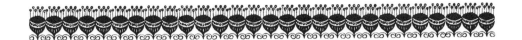

# CONTENTS

# Part 3    Between Two Worlds

# Part 4    Luke

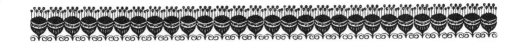

# FOREWORD

*Philip R. A. May, M.D.**

Trudi Schoop brings profound insight, pungent description, and a highly personal style to the depiction of bodily expression and existence and to the understanding and psychotherapeutic management of the schizophrenic condition.

In 1958, when she first described to me the conceptual basis of her approach, I was much intrigued and I recognized that these ideas were very much in tune with modern dynamic psychology. In the final analysis, the body ego and its mental representation, the body image, are the fundamental basis for human relationships and they play a central role in determining our perceptions of reality. Indeed, dissolution of ego boundaries, and of relationships between "self" and "not-self," and unrealistic concepts of what is good and bad about the self and others are now widely held to be basic disturbances in schizophrenia.

*Professor of Psychiatry in Residence, Neuropsychiatric Institute, California State Department of Mental Hygiene and University of California at Los Angeles; Chief of Staff for Program Evaluation, Research and Education, Veterans Administration Hospital, Brentwood, California.

I was so impressed by this correspondence with psycho-dynamic theory that I naively asked which of the distinguished Swiss clinicians had given her these very sophisticated ideas. In retrospect, I think she must have discerned some appearance of good intent, or at least a readiness to learn, underneath my habitual tendency to move speedily and with concerned concentration into almost any subject. At any rate, I was graciously and with humor acquainted with the fact that posture, gesture, movement, body image, identity, non-verbal communication, identification, and projection of the self are the basic sciences of the dancer. Apparently, I discovered, a dancer's professional life requires studying the body just as others study the mind.

I was Clinical Director and Chief of Research at Camarillo Hospital in those days and I was convinced that I had come across something that had exciting promise as a hitherto untapped, largely non-verbal approach for research and development in dynamic psychology—particularly the understanding and treatment of the schizophrenic patient. So, I decided then and there to convert Trudi as far into research as we could go. It turned out that the main difficulty was not Trudi's conversion, but convincing the psychiatric research system that this was serious research and not an artistic boondoggle. It is an unfortunate fact that our research system was, and still is, geared to the orderly support of certain types of highly structured academic and laboratory research. When it comes to developing novel and somewhat intangible clinical ideas that are still in the exploratory phase, you might as well try to sell the system the Brooklyn Bridge.

Happily, with some assistance from the California State Department of Mental Hygiene and through interested private individuals, we did manage to develop some research ventures and in general, they prospered. We were able to show in a controlled scientific study that the approach had potential with very sick schizophrenic patients, not as a cure-all, but in making contact and establishing a relationship and in preparing the way for other forms of therapy such as psychotherapy and sociotherapy.

We didn't actually make a formal study of the interaction between a body-ego approach and use of tranquilizing drugs, but I think we know enough to give a reasonably firm answer.

On the one hand, in high doses, these drugs may have Parkinson-like side effects—shakiness, stiffness, and emotional unresponsiveness—that must not only affect the body image and sense of self, but also restrict the patient's range and capability of movement. On the other hand, they greatly reduce psychotic thought disorder and improve communication, so that the patients previously unwilling or unable to cooperate can enter into a meaningful relationship. The two methods of treatment—drug therapy and body ego—should not stand in opposition, or in competition as replacements for each other. On the contrary, the discerning therapist will use them together in whatever combination and timing will most effectively liberate the patient from his psychosis. Thus the proper application of Trudi Schoop's methods will require close and sensitive integration with drug therapy. Dosage must be adjusted in an informed manner, continually in tune with the patient's progress, as close as possible to the ideal where the patient is given enough medication to counteract the disturbance of thought process and ability to enter into a relationship, yet not too much so that he is sleepy, stiff, or unresponsive. Similarly, non-verbal and verbal therapy should be seen as complementary and potentially concurrent approaches, not as mutually exclusive or in conflict. Body-ego methods can be more than a preliminary to verbal contact: they have been used successfully in combination with verbal psychotherapy.

Even more important, we were able to work through ideas and concepts and to help Trudi to systematize and formalize them into a technique that could be used with patients and taught to other therapists. It gives me particular pleasure that she has now written down in her book her philosophy and understanding of the personal non-verbal messages radiated by the body and the concepts of her therapeutic approach, so that others may learn and be encouraged to experiment and develop along these lines. It is a unique contribution to the clinical literature on schizophrenia, as well as to the field of dance.

As I read through the manuscript, I was struck by the parallel between the verbal and non-verbal therapeutic process in schizophrenia, on the one hand, and the requirements for successful therapists in both modes, on the other. In fact, I realized that it had enabled me to identify and formulate more clearly my own ideas about the characteristics of those therapists who seem to be particularly gifted in working with schizophrenic patients.

It seems to me that, more important than mere technical training and length of experience or mealy-mouthed clichés such as warmth and understanding, are a deeply ingrained and heightened sense and valuation of inner and outer freedom, not as a political issue, but as a fundamental human concern; a sincere affection and tolerance for human foibles; a profound respect for each person's uniqueness. And a good humored acceptance of one's own fallability—the therapist cannot afford to be always right in this business. Such therapists see the patient, not as a psychiatric case, but, to use Trudi's phrase, as a "fascinating foreigner." They enjoy and respond to the challenge of penetrating his idiosyncratic personal language and entering into his country and customs, of seeing and feeling the world as he does.

Trudi's observation that the schizophrenic plays out, in his own personal theatre, fragments of comedy, slapstick, and tragedy leads me to realize that the gifted therapists of my acquaintance are all, in their own way, superb actors—and they are well aware that they are on stage when they enter the hospital wards. I would therefore speculate that the task for the therapist is to enter the patient's private stage and to dramatize and simplify reality for him—and perhaps also for his family and the ward staff.

He must project an image of himself that is natural and direct, larger than life. In this way, the schizophrenic is provided with a magnified external object with whom he can identify and against which his projections can be tested. The play is not always high drama. The gifted therapist frequently softens his interpretations and confrontations with the elements of comedy, in the sense of portraying an affectionate and amusing, non-hostile image of the patient and of those around him. And, following Bleuler, he dares at times to surprise and shock his patients a little—as Linda was shaken by being tricked into recognizing that her face was a part of her being.

We are shown in this book how the elements of dance can be used to meet and accept the schizophrenic the way he is. In an atmosphere of freedom to make his own investigations, the patient is helped to examine and comprehend the good and the bad in himself, and to review his own development. Then the task is to point out the possibilities of change, while never cutting off his freedom to return to his own original pattern. And in the final stage, when he has developed understanding and a movement vocabulary, he is ready to explore spontaneous action, to search for authentic self, to gain a freedom to act as he feels and to communicate this to others.

It is well that at critical points in the text Trudi places "dance" and "dancers" in inverted commas. "Dancing" to her is not a matter of prowess and technique: it is a personally created style of physical movement that projects a person's being, not the execution of preconceived dance combinations. In fact, we learn that technique can be used as an intellectualizing defense against understanding of the self.

In the non-verbal mode, as in formal psychotherapy, we see that immense patience may be required in the laborious and time-consuming attempt ". . . sensitively to intrude upon such monumental privacy." We are shown how delusions may be portrayed and explored in movement, as a mode of entry into the psychotic world, as a way to dramatize their contrast with reality. This process is described in a vivid language of movement that contrasts with the drab technicalities of psychotherapy literature: ". . . Rather than suppressing the fantasy of a psychotic individual, we should fly with him for a while, then descend with him for a soft landing on this earth. In giving shape to his visions, he will create a work that fuses fantasy and reality." And we see the value of daring to imitate the patients' behavior, even of purposefully caricaturing and parodying his splits and mechanisms as a prelude to re-integration.

It would be, I think, a misinterpretation to apply a rigorous distinction between mind and body, between verbal and non-verbal—Trudi herself emphasizes their close identity by the terms "motionally" and "emotionally." While Trudi paced silently with Mary for months, there was a continuing sequence of unspoken transactions at a number of levels. When Mary finally spoke, she did not perceive it as strange that she should speak—the transactions had merely shifted to another language. Commands to the physical body were to Henry an analog of psychological relationships with his wife. Differences in the rhythm of beaters may be a metaphor for agreement and disagreement.

As Leopold Bellak, in *Schizophrenic Syndrome*, observed about the work of Madame Sechchayes: meticulous, laborious, loving, carefully thought-out rebuilding of a severely defective personality may be impractical for the millions of schizophrenics in the world, yet exceedingly valuable for learning from the few to the many. And so it is with the work of Trudi Schoop. It may lead, in the long run, to treatment methods that can be used in earlier as well as in later stages of the illness and with larger numbers of patients. It has already taken a giant step in this direction.

WON'T YOU JOIN THE DANCE?

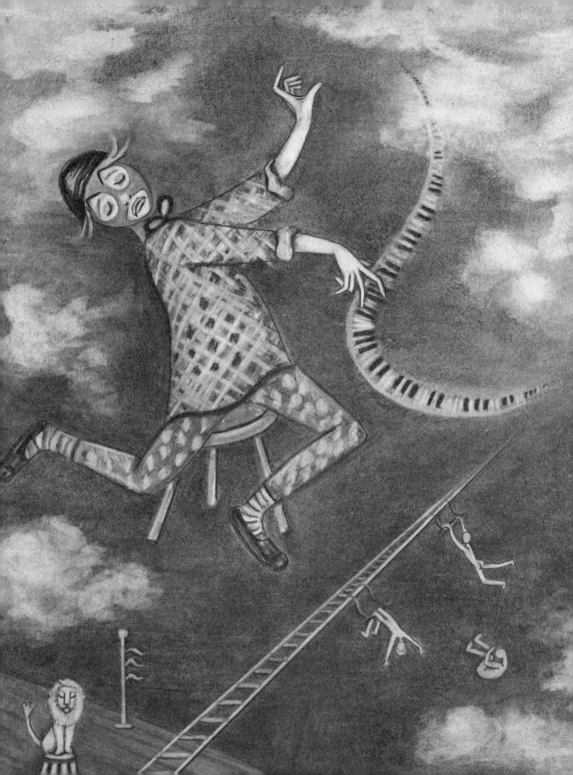

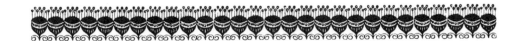

# PROLOGUE
## Stage One

**Trudi**

Whenever I think back to my childhood, feelings of boundless gratitude and happiness come over me. Ours was a Swiss family, ruled with a non-iron hand by Father, a man respected and appreciated by Zurich's intellectuals, and by Mother, a warm and loving woman with an almost insatiable urge for freedom. My mother recognized no moralistic taboos, followed no conventional rules. She just did what seemed right for her. My father loved her dearly and admired her inner strength and free spirit; it was she who set the liberated climate in our household. A strong and courageous man himself, my father was the editor of a Zurich newspaper and president of the beautiful Dolder Hotels. Such a man should probably have led the decorous life expected of him by the quite bourgeois society of that lovely, ancient city on the Lake of Zurich. But he would not. He loved my unruly mother so much that, rather than try to tame her, he supported her offbeat ways and wishes.

I remember vividly our dinner table, which was really more like a conference table—with wild discussions, very much to eat, and so many people that we children often sat on the floor. There were Mother and Father and the four children, each of us usually having brought along at least one friend. Sharing the meal with us were Lisi, our beloved cook with the big bosom and the ever-friendly face, and two young maids from the French part of Switzerland, who spoke only French and were terribly homesick. There were usually some business friends of my father's and at least three or four struggling writers or actors or painters, a young priest from Italy, a communist from Russia, and a baroness from Germany . . . all surviving their dark days together in my mother's generous house.

And I remember the excitement when my father brought some sandals home and announced that he intended to wear them without socks! And I can still see my mother throwing her corset away one day, and recall how she began to wear colorful, loose-fitting clothes and to look with pity at all the ladies with their suffering waistlines. And, of course, all her children had to be colorfully and comfortably dressed, too. I'm sure we looked like the forerunners of a little hippy colony, and that was much for Zurich to swallow. We were probably accepted as the Swiss family that proved to be the exception to the rule!

There was my brother Max, who was to become a painter, and my brother Paul, who would be a composer-pianist and write the scores for my pantomimes, and my sister Hedi, who would excel as a dancer, actress, ceramist, painter—and who now, of course, illustrates this book. The four of us lived wildly in our beautiful house on the hills above Zurich. Summer after summer I lived in a tree-house I'd built in one of the huge oaks that dominated our immense garden. I was never asked to sleep "for-heaven's-sake-in-the-house" or in my own bed. My parents were happy to see me whenever I appeared for the family meals, to which I made impressive entrances, looking like one of the gnomes from A Midsummer Night's Dream. Only when my food supply ran low did I come down from my tree-house—or when I, myself, strongly felt the need for a hot bath!

Those summers were just heavenly. Our home grounds must

have looked like a Garden of Eden Annex with our four naked young bodies rolling in the high grass, climbing trees to break fruit from their branches, and followed, wherever we played, by cats and dogs and tame crows and not-so-tame mountain goats.

School, of course, was a different chapter in our young lives. It was hard for us to adjust to the stern discipline of a dehumanized system and to be shut up in a classroom where children had to sit still, where nobody was interested in how they felt, and where the best scholar was the one who could somehow manage to divorce his head from the rest of his body and thereby facilely count, multiply, solve algebra problems, memorize history and long, boring poetry.

When I once aired my gripes against the academic life to my mother, she said, "Don't worry. Anything you don't need to know for the life you choose, you will forget the minute you get out of school."

And that's just what I did—thoroughly! Perhaps my father was disappointed. I think he would have loved me to be a teacher, as he had been in his youth. Actually he was the last in a long ancestral line of scholars, professors, and instructors that can be traced way back to the time of our beloved and idealistic Pestalozzi, the man who founded a home and school for war orphans when Switzerland was fighting for its freedom.

At the age of twelve I was firmly resolved to become an actress. While still in school I studied with ingenuous enthusiasm the great dramatic parts of world literature. My drama teacher was delighted with my talent. Up to this day I don't know why, because I didn't understand a single line I spoke, let alone the spiritual content of the dramas.

One thing I know for sure: the more horror there was, the more heads rolled, the more blood gushed, the more injustice fell upon the innocent, the more satisfaction I derived from my role. For two years I learned without learning, understood without understanding. Then suddenly a change occurred. I wanted to dance. I wanted to express my own ideas and my own feelings through my body and not through words I did not comprehend. I sat up in my tree-house and thought about it very hard. Then, one evening at the dinner table, I stood up and announced that

I had come to a very important decision: I was going to be a dancer. The response was overwhelming. Family and friends roared with such laughter that I couldn't continue my carefully planned speech. Finally, my mother came to my rescue.

"Don't be so ridiculous," she scolded them. "I think it's just wonderful that Trudi knows what she wants. Let's give her a chance to prove it." And she looked long at my father.

So at the age of sixteen, I tried to create dances. I had had no training; I didn't know how to go about making a dance. But I did make dances. I rented a big room, hired a piano player, had ideas, searched for music, rehearsed and trained according to a do-it-yourself system, designed highly complicated costumes, neglected food and sleep, and was immensely happy despite all the difficulties I was running into.

If ever there was a time when body and spirit separated, it happened to me at that period of my life. I longed to be wondrously beautiful, ethereal, and harmonious, but my sturdy legs stood crooked, I stumbled over my feet, my body was heavy and its movements contorted with yearning. It was, to put it mildly, a heroic struggle between spirit and matter.

From the chaos of my ideas and my cumbersome body there gradually emerged more or less discernible shapes of dances. These dances, though childlike, were intended to be deadly serious: A white flower opening to the light of the sun in order to fall asleep in the evening. A crow stalking in the field, polishing its feathers. A sad little girl crying because she is alone. A beautiful lady snakecharmer. And above all, a slave with chained hands rebelling against his fate. This last dance was my pride and joy; it embodied my longing for inner and outer freedom.

Also, I simply interpreted music, such as Liszt's "Grand Gallope," whose speed I could never keep up with, and Schubert's "Moments Musicales," whose playfulness contrasted grotesquely with my earthbound body. I shortened or arranged classical and modern music to fit my purpose and crudely eliminated whatever I was not able to master, either technically or emotionally.

And when, about six months later, I gave my first dance recital, it was, believe it or not, a smashing success. The critics raved, my father was proud, and my mother smiled. My triumph was understandable only as a reflection of the mood of the time. When I started to dance, the dancers of Europe (particularly Germany) were just beginning to reach for new contents and forms. Down with ballet, down with sweet loveliness! The best people were against classical form, against tradition, against anything, in any case. The Weisenthal sisters had thrown their ballet slippers into a corner and danced with bare feet. Isadora Duncan preached natural movement, the flowing line. The tutu was replaced by a sort of Greek tunica. Rudolf von Laban began to classify dancers into three categories: high, medium, and low. And he was devoted to what he called *Ausdruckstanz* (Expression-Dance), which was new and almost frightening. Emile Jacques-Dalcroze tried to integrate completely music and movement. Mary Wigman danced without music. She believed in dance as an independent art that could speak for itself. Valeska Gert, on the other hand, accompanied her dances with words and yells. In her chalk-white makeup she looked like a poster by Toulouse Lautrec.

All this was exciting, new, oppositional. Everywhere things were on the move. Everybody tried to be original, daring. In the beginnings of modern dance, opposition against tradition was of the essence. Representative technique had not yet been developed. Anyone who thought he had something to say, and who possessed two legs, danced. The theatres were swamped with dance recitals. Names by the hundreds flared up in the stage firmament and faded away. One stamped and screamed on stage, one mimicked madness with a flower in hand. One danced morphine in a long purple gown and a pale green face. One danced vice itself with a long cigarette holder. On red couches, rapes and murders were committed in dance. All this was expressed in crude movements, and often without any effort to be understood. The leaps ended with a thud; the stages thundered under the impact of falling bodies. The corps de ballet was replaced by the *Bewegungschöre* (movement choir). Janitors, housewives, secretaries, clerks, policemen, and physicians streamed into these groups and expressed their joint feelings in joint movements. Soon opera was using the *Bewegungschöre* for big mass scenes, preferably the ones playing in hell, where devils of both sexes jumped horrifyingly about. It was very strange. When I came to Germany from Switzerland I gained the impression that all the Germans were dancing.

It was at this time that I began to train seriously for the dance. I had proved to myself and my environment that I wanted to be a dancer; now I had to turn my body into a capable instrument, choosing ballet for my technical training. Simultaneously, I attended the school of Ellen Tells, a disciple of Isadora Duncan. She taught the expression of pure and nobly flowing movements. Lacking easy grace, I suffered from my leadenness, and the inexorable rigidity of ballet was bodily punishment for me.

During this period of study, I toured Germany and Switzerland. I danced in sold-out theatres with great, very great success. The audience went wild with enthusiasm and the critics sang my praises. Why, then, was it that such response impressed me so little? I had outgrown my childhood dances. Now I had to find a way to express the "current me."

It was at this time that, suddenly and unexpectedly, my father died. His death shook me to the roots of my being. My world had always depended on him for moral support, now I was determined to be self-reliant. I decided to open a school for "artistic dancing." The city of Zurich gave me one of the most beautiful small old churches to use as a dance studio. There was just one string attached: I had to wind the steeple clock to keep the neighborhood informed of the time! . . . The time often stood still, but not the telephone, which jangled with calls from infuriated citizens.

During this hiatus I worked with many, many pupils and became acquainted with a new aspect of life. Teaching so fascinated me that I became completely immersed in my new task, placing my choreographic development in the background for the time being. The hours I spent watching the movements of my pupils were periods of intense reverence. The pupils seemed to be approaching creation, as movement developed from movement, as they strove for form, for choreographic expression of an idea. But at the same time I began to realize how difficult it was for them to express their fantasies, to "move their imaginations." Personal affectations, feelings of inferiority and anxiety, conflicts of all sorts hemmed in their bodies and cramped their actions. I had begun to see people in a new light.

On the streets I followed strangers, imitating their gait and posture, and imagined, by taking in their manner of movement, that I was able to feel their state of mind. Suddenly I was obsessed with human gestures, with the play of features, with attitude and countenance, with the sparkling variety of man's presence.

I was fascinated by the way a face distorted in anger, by the way someone cried, by the way someone lustily slapped his thighs. A lady checking her coiffure in the mirror, a man looking for a cuff link, a waiter waiting for a tip, a businessman talking his client into a deal—all such commonplace scenes captivated me and made me aware of the colorful eloquence of everyday life.

Again I worked on dances. This time they were different. I tried to stylize the little stories I had observed, and at the same time give them a broader, more general application. I wanted to do this, not by acting, but by telling my stories with my body, by dancing them. They had to be short, and so precise that it was next to impossible to find the right music for them. But one day, my brother Paul sat down with me and began to translate my ideas into musical sequences. I had found my composer!

The new dances were entitled: *You Interest Me, Business Is Business, It Was Only a Pain, Nothing More, I Like Myself, The Big NO!, The Art of Free Speech*. And the first time I made my appearance with this program, I had the shock of my life. The audience laughed! That had never happened to me before. I had composed those dances with utmost seriousness. Not for a minute had I intended to be funny. But that night I learned from the audience that I was a "comic" dancer.

In the late twenties I found myself in Berlin, performing in a little avant-garde cabaret, Die Katakombe. Here, I joined a group of several young actors, musicians, and a writer, all of whom wanted a political stage. The oncoming nightmare of another war could already be felt in the air. We had a target for our criticism. We made fun of the self-satisfied bourgeoisie, and satirized the arrogance of the emerging "Master Race." Whatever we did was young, blunt, and terribly cocky. But there was nothing chaotic or indecipherable about our statements, as there had been when the artistic revolution first began. We wanted to formulate clearly. We wanted to be unmistakably understood. Together, we found a daring form to present a daring content. The little political show triumphed and, for the first time, I felt that my personal success was deserved. I had applied my talent to serve a cause and found out that dance can be an incisive weapon.

While I worked with this group, I was still performing as a soloist. If I wanted a partner, I had to address myself to an imaginary one. I remember dancing *Promenade with a Friend* and wishing that my invisible listener were real. More and more, I wanted a dialogical situation. I wanted to people the stage with other characters so that together we could show how man deals with man: How do people love, hate, dupe each other? How do they play together? What do they gossip about? Rejoice in? Grieve over?

I was absorbed in such reflections when I was invited to participate in the International Dance Congress in Paris. I accepted, and formed a group with my best pupils. Though they were non-professionals, each one was talented and each one eager. I already had a pantomime in mind in which dancing and acting would be integrated. It was the dance-comedy *Fridolin*. As Fridolin, I played a naive youngster, full of dreams, who could not adjust to his narrow, materialistic world. Somehow this awkward, comical figure represented my own conflict with society as I saw it. I was one of the prize-winners at the Paris congress. The critics went overboard in their praise. I can still recall the thrill of standing in the lobby the next morning, reading their reviews. "The elementary art of dance receives new meaning; first in *The Green Table* by Kurt Joos: the peace message against war, then with Trudi Schoop: the message of humanity in our time. Here the pathos of Joos, there the mocking aggressiveness of Trudi Schoop."

I had found my way—and very soon after, a husband! And until this day, I believe that he fell as much in love with my talent as he did with my person. He certainly helped me in every way possible to realize my professional dreams. With his assistance, I was now able to assemble a group of professional dancers. It was a motley company, as different as can be imagined in character, appearance, technique, and nationality. I engaged acrobats with no dance training, musical comedy performers, ballet girls, and specialty dancers. It wasn't easy to weld that heterogeneous group into a performing unit. The dancers didn't want to act, the actors didn't want to dance, the acrobats insisted on standing on their heads all the time, the modern dancers hated the ballet people, and the ballet people sneered at modern dance. And all of them distrusted my new ideas of comical pantomime. But at last they came around, each one's individual expression making a vital contribution to the whole.

My dreams about the group had come true. Many programs came into being in the course of the years: *Fridolin en Route* and *Fridolin at Home, Want Ads, Ringelreihen, Blonde Marie, In the Name of Love, Barbara.* All the pantomimes were humorous statements about man's imperfections. Though they ridiculed, they were somehow affectionately tolerant. Each program was a full feature—one comedy in two or three acts—and most of the productions were made in musical collaboration with my brother Paul.

For several gratifying years I travelled all over the world with my group of twenty dancers and two pianists. And I'll never forget our whispered, backstage excitement one opening night in Prague, when we learned that the great Sol Hurok was in the audience. What a celebration followed his offer to book us for a tour in America! And, once across the Atlantic, we really covered territory: up and down and across this huge land we travelled, principally by bus. I think we played every major city. Little did I know, when we performed in Los Angeles, that I'd someday be a confirmed California resident.

We were in the mid-Atlantic, after our fifth American visit, when the war broke out. My group disbanded, each member hurrying to return to his own country. Hedi had long ago fled to America with her husband, Friederich Hollaender, and my mother and brothers had already joined her there.

Switzerland was like the eye of a hurricane, surrounded on all sides by the raging war-storm. I involved myself in Red Cross work, helping to care for the trainloads of mutilated soldiers that

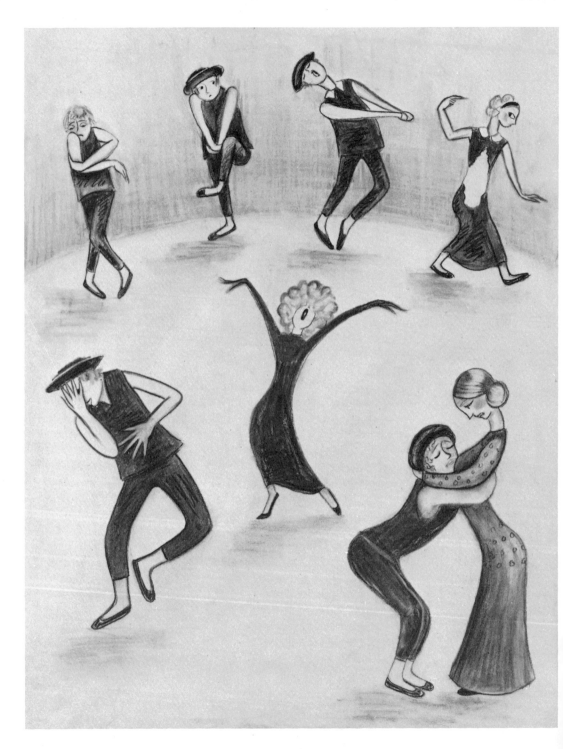

passed through our neutral land. At the Pestalozzidorf, I worked and played and danced with the little orphans who had somehow made their way out of the holocaust and into that idyllic refuge.

Eventually I joined another political cabaret. What the Katakombe had been for Germany fifteen years before, the Cornichon was now for Switzerland. Through the Cornichon, Switzerland could air its distress about Hitler's Germany, and we, the Cornichon, could criticize our own government for its indifference to the plight of our neighbor-countries and for its inconsiderate treatment of the refugees who crossed our borders. In spite of our open accusations, the government stood steadfastly beside us. The Swiss censor often let us know in advance when the German consul or press attaché was going to visit the cabaret. We could then alter our own material accordingly. It was a fearfully exciting time, a time of never knowing what we could say and what we could not—or even if we'd be able to perform at all. Gradually we constructed a secret vocabulary, a kind of sign language, that defied censorship. The Germans could hardly report, "Trudi Schoop draped her fingers over her brow. We feel that she was making fun of Hitler's forelock!" Our cast included singers, writers, painters, dancers—each tops in his own field, and all united in a keen effort to fight with our art for our beliefs. Throughout this horrible period, when the bombers flew nightly over darkened Zurich, we sang, played, and danced our political messages to packed houses.

As the Germans marched relentlessly through Europe, my wishful fantasy led me to dance Hitler as "The Dying Swan." A black tutu suggested the uniform of the SS and my face was adorned with a mustache like the Führer's. The last movements of my expiring swan were a series of frenzied salutes: the "wing" was stiffly raised over and over again until this macabre bird fell dead! I performed that satire only once. The German consul was outraged and my own government decidedly nervous.

**Trudi**

At length, the terrible war drew to a close. The Cornichon had served its purpose. There was another tour with my group through Europe and America. I was still in the United States when word came that my husband had died. . . .

There followed a period of emptiness. I was tired of moving

# Part 1

# THE DOOR WITHOUT A HANDLE

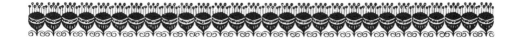

# CONFRONTATION

## "Ah Sish Aristo Shah!"

It was a beautiful morning for driving up the valley to the state hospital. The mustard was in full bloom that day, wrapping the soft, rounded hills in golds of every hue, under a sky that stretched silky-blue from horizon to horizon. How I love this sun-drunken country where the ocean's fluid rhythm seems to extend into the landscape. My car roller-coasted smoothly up and down the earth-waves, passing sleek horses and wide-eyed cattle wandering through pastures splashed with blue lupine.

My body shifted slightly, telling me that I'd been sitting in one frozen position ever since I'd left home: hands clutching the steering wheel like a vise, shoulders hiked up, neck so stiff that it crackled when I moved it. Why all this tension? What's the matter with me anyway? . . . I know, I know, . . . it's that letter, lying open on the seat beside me. How ridiculous to be so scared of it! Nobody forced me into this situation; I *asked* for that letter. I wrote them first. I wanted to work with their patients. Of course,

I *could* call the whole thing off . . . I could play sick . . . or say that I have to go suddenly back to Switzerland . . . I can turn around right now!

A road sign appeared over the next rise: NO U TURN. Oh well, the doctors just want to talk to me; that's their right. It's really a very nice letter. ". . . Thank you for offering your services. . . . Dance Therapy sounds interesting . . . would like to hear more about your method . . . meet with us Wednesday, 10 A.M." And here it is Wednesday, 9:30 A.M. I'd better hurry up. If my hands would only stop that "stage-fright itching"! Why didn't I apply at a nice, small, private hospital? Any kind of state institution scares me. They're all so impersonal, so academic! But in a hospital this size, there's sure to be a greater variety of patients. How vividly I remember Professor Bleuler's patients in Zurich when, many years ago, he asked me to perform for them. How black and white were their expressions—without any shading—only angry, only fearful, only. . . . My heart quickened in anticipation. Would the patients be the same in this country, in this hospital? And what would I do with them if they were? I didn't know. Any ideas I did have were still in a dream stage. The doctors certainly don't need my dreams; they need facts, results, and, right now, a description of my method. Can I ever admit my hope to learn from the patients themselves as I seek to establish a clear-cut working method? All I know is that somehow I want to dance with them. Dance? In a hospital? With psychotic patients? At this point, the idea seems absurd even to me. But why, I wonder? Does the word "dance" still connote exhibitionism, narcissism, depravity? Is dancing just too pleasurable to be taken seriously, too unscientific to be considered therapeutic?

My apprehension accelerated with the speedometer. Why do I put myself through this ordeal? Why is it so vitally imperative for me to become involved with people who are mentally ill? I thought again of Bleuler's patients, saw their unusual mannerisms, their weird actions, heard their strange speech patterns. **Fields of stock** What wouldn't I give to be able to understand what they're thinking, feeling, saying! So that was it, then. My infatuation with human expression had brought me to this time, this meeting, this adventure. The world was just waiting for me to decipher the

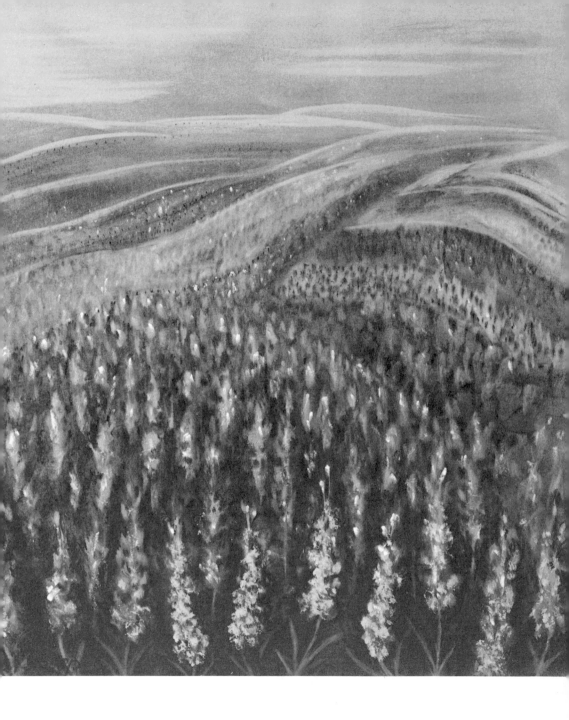

enigmatic expression of schizophrenia. Why do I have to be so expression-crazy?

I was awakened from the anxiety of reality by a dream of scent, a fantasy of perfume. Fields of stock, the flower of my childhood garden, fat, delicate, rainbow-colored stock, spread out before my enchanted eyes. Swelling, falling, overturning they radiated iridescent hues far and wide, fusing the heavens with the earth. Enraptured, I was carried away on a cloud of delight, which deposited me gently in front of the hospital. ADMINIS-TRATION, the sign said. I entered.

With the expiring hiss of a punctured balloon, the door closed itself behind me. I found myself in a darkish, colorless reception room. The air reeked of disinfectants which failed to cover up what they should have covered up! Behind the information desk, a stiff-backed woman talked on the phone in a clipped, efficient tone.

"Yes, doctor, I'll send her up when she . . . ."

Glancing over, she saw me standing respectfully a few feet away.

"Miss Schoop?" she asked, with the severity of Fräulein Bachtold, my seventh-grade teacher.

I nodded, feeling somehow guilty.

"She's just come in, Doctor Keermuschel. . . . Yes, sir, right away."

When the receiver had been neatly replaced, her curious eyes behind thick-lensed glasses gave me a quick up-and-down look of appraisal. The verdict seemed to be "how very odd!"

She spewed out directions in a steady stream: "Your meeting is in the conference room, up-the-stairs-second-floor-first-right-third-left-around-the-corner-other-side-of-a-blood-bank-laboratory-the-fourth-door-with-no-handle."

"Thank-you-very-much," my voice said as my mind struggled to cope with the floor plan.

As I climbed the stairs, my heartbeat hammered in my throat, tripling the tempo of my steps. What will I say? How will I say it? I'll never be able to explain in English what I want to do. Don't fool yourself—you can't even explain it in Swiss!

I reached the second floor and took the first right.

18

Oh God, and what will I ever do without "okay"? My sister just said yesterday that the way I used "okay" showed a low grade of education. I *could not* use it with the doctors. Unfortunately, it was the one, single word I could say with confidence . . . in front of a sentence, in the middle of a sentence, and at the end. Besides, it was my delaying device; it gave me time to think. And it could mean just about anything! What a shame that this wonderful term, the only one I could pronounce decently in American English, was *out.*

I found myself in a dead-end corridor and retraced my steps for a new start. How in the world will I ever talk to them? Maybe it will be okay if I say, "I believe in the body as a partner of the mind. I would like to make your patients feel better and I think I could do it with movements. I would work for a body that likes to express itself very strong, very throofully . . . throughfully? . . . troofully?" As I wondered how the real Americans would spell this difficult word, I passed the blood bank and found the fourth door. She was right. It had no handle!

I took a deep breath and summoned my life-long defense against authority. A "charming, ingenuous child" knocked at the door. It opened to admit me . . . Dr. Keermuschel, Hospital Director, very courteous, very blue-eyed.

Three minutes later, the dreaded interview was over. But within that tiny fraction of time, the coin of my life flipped over. Dazedly, I remembered Dr. Keermuschel introducing me to a cluster of disinterested faces.

"My colleagues," he said, gesturing courteously toward six men who for 180 seconds managed to remain mute.

Then came The Question: "Well, Miss Schoop. What can you do for us? We'd like to know something about your method, how you go about it, and what makes you think it would work. Just what do you plan to do with the patients?

Words came out of my mouth heedlessly, earnestly: "Okay. I would like to dance with your patients, okay?"

Utter silence. The doctor's gaze—a blue laser beam searching my soul . . .

"OKAY!" With this one glorious word he made me a dance therapist.

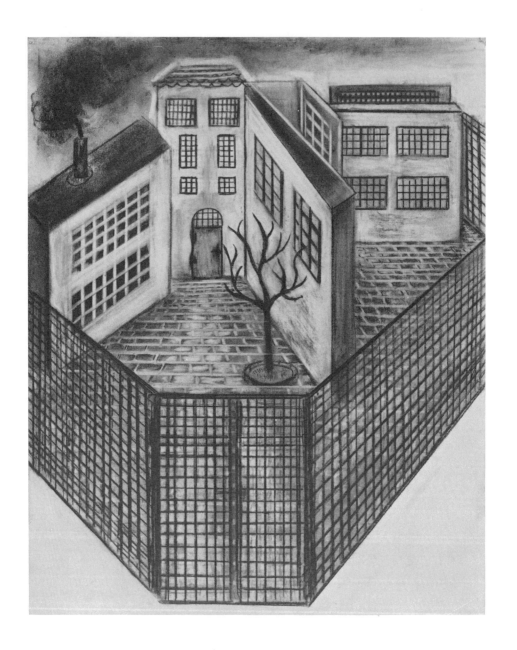

More words, only dimly recorded by my ears. ". . . saw you perform in Chicago . . . your pantomimes . . . an instinctive understanding of human behavior . . . interesting to see how you'd apply this therapeutically . . . innovative approach to treatment . . ."

Then: "Goodbye . . . good luck . . . Dr. Benson will show you around. . . ."

Miracle concluded. I was going to be allowed to dance with patients. Right here, in this hospital. The young man beside me was taking me to visit the wards. Stunned and elated, I followed him down the hall and the tour began. We walked through interminable corridors, separated one from another by forbidding iron gates. The silence was broken only by the sound of our footsteps and the clattering of keys as my guide unlocked each barrier for us to pass through, and then relocked it. This procedure was carried out in a carefully rehearsed and exactly timed pattern, a ritual with a purpose unknown to me. I began to feel that we were travelling through a strange dream, leaving our world farther and farther behind us as gate after gate closed at our backs. At last we faced a solid, massive door. No sound penetrated from the other side. Like Bluebeard's wife, torn between curiosity and dread, I waited for the last key to be fitted and turned. The door was flung open. I stepped over the threshold.

My eyes blinked in the sudden sunlight that blazed through long, barred windows . . . more bars at the door leading to a barred courtyard . . . everywhere, bars. I faced the people whose difference those bars respected and protected. There sat an old man, head tilted grotesquely toward his right shoulder, motionless. An emaciated girl huddled on the floor, rocking desperately in never-ending repetition. A grinning woman, her back pressed close to the wall, invited me with upraised fists to box with her: "Wanna fight? Wanna fight?" Along the right side of the room, a man marched with military precision, eight steps left, about-face; eight steps right, about-face; again and again and again. I saw a lined face, like a classic mask of tragedy, superimposed upon a body that gaily skipped and flitted about the ward. Another being crawled on the floor, searching . . . anxiously searching . . . only searching. And under a light fixture a young man, deep in conversation with an electric bulb. The room was

**Everywhere bars**

filled with mirthless giggling, occasional sobs, sudden shouts, aimless chatter, monotonous movement: a photomontage of sight and sound. Amid the churning confusion, transfixed in stillness, were the living statues; bodies seemingly tossed into frozen positions. One standing immobile by a window, off-balance, arms helplessly outflung. Another sitting bolt upright on a bench, caught in irrevocable tension, eyes staring at . . .?? What went on deep within these arrested forms?

I felt a series of quick little tugs at my sleeve. A tiny child-woman, pale, moon-faced, stood on tiptoe close to my side, whispering frantically . . .

"Ah sish aristo shah!"

Nodding and shaking her head, with its cascades of hair, she peeked furtively over her shoulder.

"Shah, aristo shah!"

The secret whispering hissed through the barrier of one translucent, blue-veined hand. Each finger was adorned with a ribbon of a different color. Whoever tied all those pretty bows for her?

"Shah! Hipto shah! Ra-ta-shah!"

"HEAR WHAT THE SPIRIT SAITH UNTO THE CHURCHES!" A Gothic figure from a stained-glass window stood before me—tall, gaunt, arms outstretched. The man's cavernous eyes stared out from hidden recesses, piercing through mine and far beyond.

"AS MANY AS I LOVE, I REBUKE AND CHASTEN!" One arm stretched high, forefinger pointing to a vengeful God-in-Heaven. "BE ZEALOUS, THEREFORE, AND REPENT!"

A bouncing cherub of a man burst in on our tightly knit threesome and took immediate control of the situation:

"Come, come, John! That's enough for today," and the evangelist was banished. "You, too, Isabel, let go of our visitor so I can show her around." He disentangled her clutching hand and drew me aside.

"Allow me to introduce myself," he suggested with a gallant bow. "My name is Andrew Carrington." His knees bounced, up-down-up-down. His fingers snapped . . . crack, crack, crack, crack! "I own this little place. Got a very good deal on it about a year ago from a fellow who lost his shirt in Vegas. Of course, it can

**Isabelle**

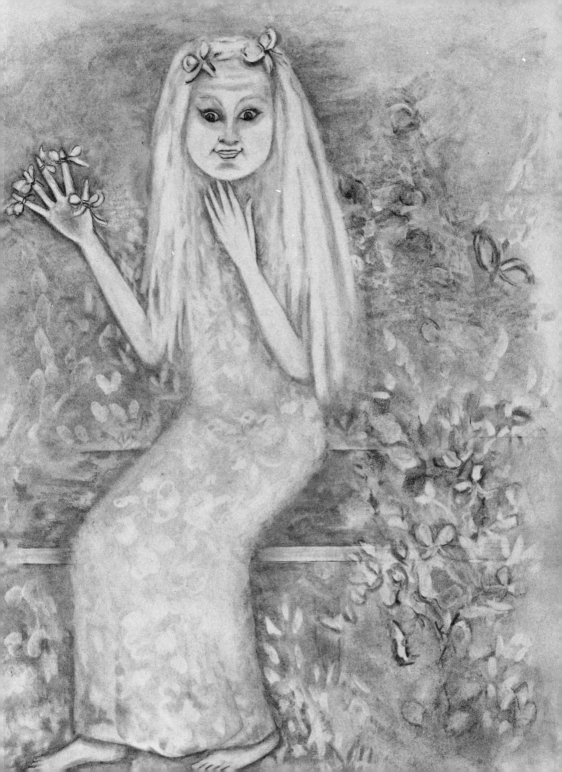

take some shaping up, but all in good time, all in good time" (. . . bounce, bounce, bounce). "Meanwhile, it has some excellent features" (. . . snap, snap, snap). "Topnotch, you might say!"

His enthusiasm was contagious. I followed the gliding bounces, the snapping fingers, as he pointed out his assets with prideful flourishes: the TV, the ping-pong table, the hard oak benches, the lone rubber tree in the center of the courtyard. Then, with the unflagging courtesy of a social director, Mr. Carrington introduced me to some of his tenants. Among them I met one Satan (round, bald, staring at his feet); two Eisenhowers: the General (saluting smartly), and the President (eyebrows raised high, in a look of permanent surprise); Marilyn Monroe (rummaging through the contents of her huge purse); and the Virgin Mary (blowing gum-bubbles, giggling when they burst).

As I was listening to Satan's lengthy dissertation on the merits of the Dodgers' baseball team, the doctor caught my eye and signalled that it was time to leave. Isabel pressed one of her ribbons into my hand. It was the pale blue one from her little finger.

While the doctor concluded his instructions to the attendants and the great door was being unlocked, I looked back once more. An atmosphere of abstraction hung over the ward, and abstracted were all the individuals living out their dream-like lives within the utilitarian dormatories and dayrooms. Spellbound, I watched the portrayals, the personifications. It seemed to me that these men and women had all the attributes and techniques of the stage at their disposal. Here were the symbolic gestures, the magnified expressions, the intensity of projection, the masks, the make-believe, the fantasy. These people played comedy, slapstick, tragedy. Most compelling of all was the clarity of form with which their characterizations were realized. The whole scene had an illusory quality, detached and suspended in time. Nightmarish: the loneliness, the isolation of the individual. Astonishing: the choreography; eighty-seven soloists, indiscriminately cast, **Ballet of delusions** each performing his own little *divertissement à la bravura*, generously giving encore after encore. A ballet of delusions. A ghostly *perpetuum mobile*.

Ten minutes later I was back in my car heading for home.

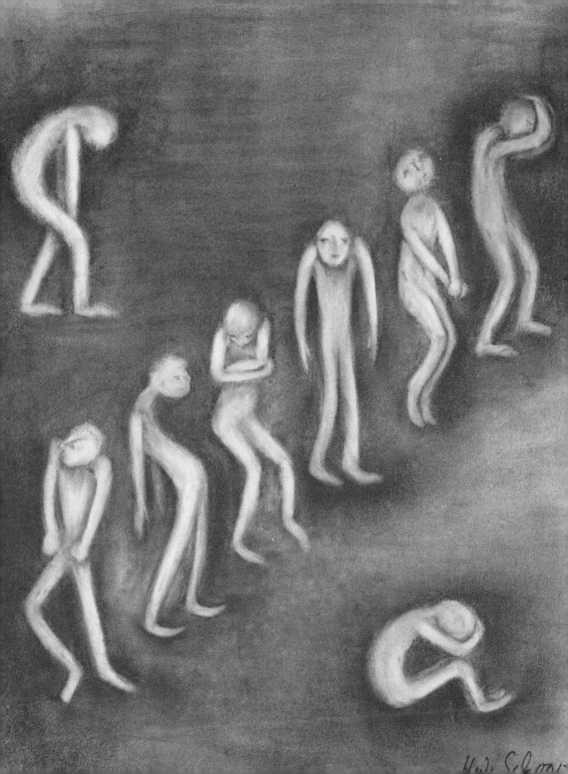

My mind was ablaze with images. It raced with questions. Would it ever be possible to meet those remote human beings on any sort of realistic level? Could I, like Pygmalion, bring the "statues" to life? . . . Oh, that's ridiculous! How could I ever? What do I know about a disturbed mind? Very, very little. Well then, what DO I know about? . . . The body, that's all. I've always thought of the body as man's tangible reality. Might not this feel-able human structure help me in my new purpose, just as well as it did during my dance career? Aside from its acquired technical skills, what else did my body contribute to that profession? Well, I certainly could always rely upon it to project an emotion, or to define a role, or to expose a character's inner self. But there was something else. . . . In the course of choreographing my fantasies and dancing them out into reality, I remember now, positive changes had occurred in my own nature. Those first pantomimes had acted as a "danced psychoanalysis" for me. Certainly my personal perspective took a turn for the better; I discovered conflicts deeply embedded, that I'd never been aware of before. . . . And now that I think of it, many of my basic problems actually disappeared. Exactly what had I done with this body of mine to create such changes? Well, I had moved it, of course, in every way I could think of, to communicate my feelings and ideas. "Communication through movement"—scarcely a revolutionary concept! There must be more to it than that; I'll have to find out. But whatever is involved in the process, it worked for me, didn't it? So isn't it feasible that it might also work for the people I visited this afternoon?

I hoped so. I wanted so desperately to try. Perhaps Isabel's ribbon would bring me luck. My fascination with this new world had begun.

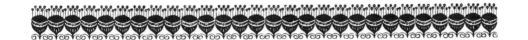

# INITIATION

# "What Ward is She From?"

MONDAY MORNING    I stood alone in the hospital's social hall, waiting for my first group of assigned patients. The doctors had trusted my ability to carry out this new program in dance therapy. Right then, I wished I could feel that same confidence. How will the patients react to the sessions? The palms of my hands were tickling again. Why must I be so nervous . . . why so afraid? There was no time to answer myself. An orderly appeared in the doorway, ushering the patients into the hall. Cautiously, they massed together near the entrance . . . waiting. . . .

"Good morning!" My cheerful tone belied my feeling. Something about the way they stood there gave me the impression that they resented having their customary routine interrupted.

"Won't you please come in?" I suggested encouragingly.

Twenty-two patients, categorized as chronic schizophrenics, gradually filtered into the room, bringing with them undercurrents of suspicion, hostility, anxiety, and mistrust. A few examined the piano. Some felt the table, touched a wall. Many circled aimlessly about, staring at the floor, and two men remained at the door, feet defiantly planted. Whatever they were doing, whether these patients were facing me or had their backs turned, I had the sensation of being furtively appraised, of undergoing an unspoken rite of initiation.

"Well, now! I would like very much to tell you who I am and why I am here. Please, will you all sit down in a circle?"

This request, which to my inexperienced mind seemed to be so natural, so simple, presented an unforeseen problem ending in disaster. Every variation of not-sitting-on-the-floor-in-a-circle unfolded before my astonished eyes. One patient draped himself over a chair. One darted across the room and started banging on the piano keys. One stooped down and hid under the table. One rolled himself up in the curtain. Some supported this organized "NO" by lying down, arguing, asking for a match, giggling, or gazing out the window. But the majority simply retreated to the security of their habitual attitudes, the long-established oblivion of their individual behavior patterns.

I made a few wretchedly unsuccessful attempts to gain their attention. Then I gave up, and concentrated on the few who were on the floor anyway. I sat down with them and began again.

"Okay! My name is Trudi. In our sessions together I will include exercises that will strengthen the muscles and make the body flexible. We will have music to dance to, and—"

"Dance!" As if on cue, there was a communal uprising. "Dance," I was told, "is for sissies." . . . "My mother wouldn't approve." . . . "Dance is against my religion." . . . And one woman announced with finality, "My aunt got measles from dancing."

In one offended body, they moved with great dignity toward the door. The orderly shrugged and began to lead them out, and through the commotion I overheard somebody's voice:

"Hey, what ward is *she* from?"

I was alone again.

TUESDAY MORNING    Again, I heard the patients shuffling down the corridor. Again, I watched them being led in by the same orderly—Mr. Dakin—who looked as tired as his group. The sight of these lackadaisical bodies confirmed my plan for the day's session.

"Today, I would like to work on feelings. Let's *show* our feelings!" I cried enthusiastically. "And let's begin with being angry. Show me how it is when you are just furious!"

The hall echoed with silence. We stared at each other for a while.

"I mean . . . show me . . . what are we *doing* when we are angry? How do we move?"

One thin voice finally broke the deadly hush: "It's not nice to be angry." A second: "I don't move when I'm angry." A third: "I'm not angry, I've never *been* angry, and I never *will* be angry!"

"Oh now, come on. It is okay to be angry. We are all angry sometimes, aren't we? I can get *very* angry!" I was beginning to feel what I said. "I, for instance, stamp my feet. I punch. I shake my fist. Like this!" And I demonstrated these symbols of wrath with all my energy and enormous affect. They liked it.

Encouraged by the first glimmer of interest, I tried to pass the ball. "Okay now! *You* be angry!"

"Do it again," someone demanded. A chorus of voices joined in, "Yeah, go on, do it again!"

So I repeated my movement study of angriness. Someone laughed. The reaction was heartening, but I knew I couldn't go on and on, entertaining twenty-two patients and an orderly. I had to do better than *that*. I had promised far more! I had to arouse their feelings! "Stamp! Punch! Hit! Cut! Box! Yell! Be angry . . . furious . . . *mad*!!" Forty-four eyes stared into faraway spaces. Forty-four arms moved helplessly. Forty-four legs tried to lift their moored feet. Twenty-two minds did not want what I wanted. Twenty-two bodies could not express what they didn't want to feel. Somebody wandered off. Somebody sat down. Somebody gazed out the window. Bored, disinterested, listless.

In despair, I again went into action. I hurled my body about in an avalanche of anger. I jumped. I hit. I raced up and down the hall. In sudden turns, I landed an attack, puffing, stamping, spitting fire; I threw myself up in the air and down on the floor in a temper tantrum. Perspiring, my heart pounding . . . I finally stopped.

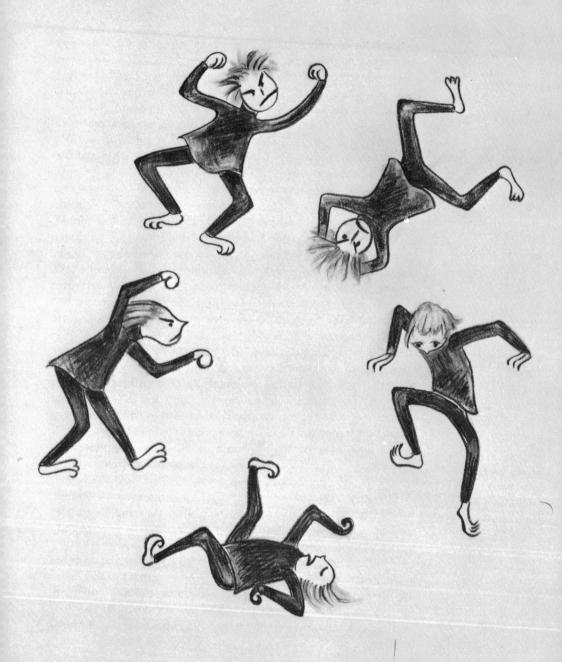

As I came to, I realized that I had lost my audience. Only two men remained on the scene. One came closer.

"Are you on bennies?" he asked.

WEDNESDAY MORNING   A little bit weak and very sore from yesterday's emotion-laden performances, I awaited my group for the third time. I felt guilty. I knew that I was the only one who had benefitted therapeutically from that session. Emptied of affect, stripped of energy, my anger was gone. Tender and loving were my sentiments this morning, toward myself, toward my patients, toward the world! It was within this all-embracing mood that I prepared to conduct today's class.

I knelt down by the piano and began to lay out my props: the reed beaters for rhythms, the colorful scarves for soft designs in space, and assortment of chimes and bells for symphonic experimentation. A cough interrupted my preparations. Standing behind me, impassively watching my actions, were the orderly and a handful of patients. I jumped to my feet, bewildered.

"Where are the others?" I asked Mr. Dakin.

"Well, it seems that there's an awful lot of sore throats going around this morning," he replied and, with a knowing wink, ambled over to his usual post by the door. For the first time, I saw him look cheerful.

Facing the remaining members of my group, I decided to begin with a beautiful swing, soft and fluid. "Let's stand in a semicircle." Their compliance was encouraging. "Now, I'd like you to swing your bodies in any way you want. Invent any kind of a swing. Let your bodies go!"

Nobody tried. I saw fear in one face, confusion in another. What had I said that was so shocking? For me, a swing is a joy. It creates such a marvelously satisfying balance between control and release.

**Avalanche of anger**

"Think of wheat fields, being blown by the wind, back and forth, up and down . . . or of ocean waves, coming in and going out!" My attempt at imagery also failed. There was no response. What had happened? What was so threatening about a free swing? Somehow, it seemed that I'd touched on dangerous territory.

31

"Look what I can do!" It was Emma. She bent over and showed me that she could touch her toes without bending her knees. Others began to touch their toes, too.

"I can do push-ups," announced Carl. And he began to demonstrate.

"When I was in the service, I used to do forty jumping-jacks without stopping!" This was Fred. "Come on," he cried, "let's do 'em! One-two-three-four, one-two-three-four!"

For the first time, I saw these individuals functioning vaguely as a group. I saw bodies moving. I saw some enthusiasm. Why did they follow Fred and not me? Gradually, the women withdrew from this strenuous masculine competition. They seated themselves close to a wall. One cried. One began to rock. Another picked her teeth.

The session was falling apart again. I *must* regain control of it somehow. At least there had been some action. Perhaps if I began by animating each body part, and strictly structured every movement . . .

"Let's see what we can do with our hands!" I called out. "We can move them up and down, side to side, around and around." A few patients started trying to follow the hand motions. "What can we do with our heads?" I continued with more assurance. "They can move up and down, side to side, and round and round and round." Except for the three isolated ones who never deviated from their own movement worlds, all the others were doing something with their heads that looked like rotation. Delighted with this success, I continued eagerly, "And what can we do with our pelvises? They can go side to side, front and back, around and ar—!"

Why did Carl stop? Why were Rosalie and Emma giggling together? What was Walter doing with his back turned? There was a shrill wolf-whistle. Fred was approaching me, his face leering suggestively, his pelvis moving back and forth in blatant sexual invitation. What if Dr. Keermuschel should come in right now? How can I handle this? I wasn't sure anymore. My confidence began to splinter. I ran for the beaters and thrust one into each person's hand.

"Let's all beat a soft waltz rhythm on the floor! Like this:

That's all for today

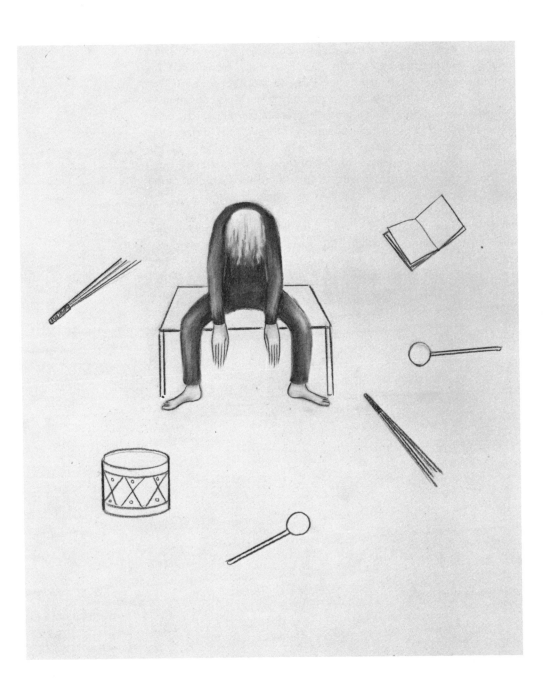

one, two, three, one, two three!" I made a last desperate effort to unify my fragmented group. But Fred only transferred his stimulated state to this new outlet. Why hit the floor when it was so much more exciting to hit the piano, the curtains, or himself? The other men picked up his lead: beaters became swords; beaters were ripped to pieces; beaters hurtled through the air; beaters chased screaming girls around the room. On the far rim of the chaos, I glimpsed the head of the orderly shaking slowly back and forth. My knees gave way. I sat down hard on the piano bench. My voice sounded faintly in my ears:

"That's all for today."

I watched our lone critic round up that turbulent group and steer them efficiently through the door. I managed to find my voice again:

"Mr. Dakin! Would you please tell Dr. Keermuschel that I won't be back until Monday? I have a very sore throat!" And I winked.

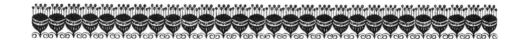

# EVALUATION

# I Save Myself a Toll Call

I began my extended weekend thinking about how miserably I had failed. What fiascos those three sessions had been! I'd just have to phone Dr. Keermuschel and tell him that he'd misplaced his trust in me, that I wasn't qualified to call myself a dance therapist.

I recalled the end of Monday's session; again I saw all the patients trooping to the door in protest. Not one had turned back to me. Not one had given me a smile. Nobody had even said goodbye. *Nobody.* Well? SO WHAT! What had I expected, for heaven's sake? That my grandiose ideas would have instantaneous success? What right had I to give in so hopelessly to my own hurt feelings? Because that was basically *it*, wasn't it? I had to be loved, accepted, admired. I could not afford to be rejected. *SISSY!*

But then . . . "Are you on bennies?" That was just the question I didn't need to hear! My exhibitionist tendencies had been discovered by a patient. Could I *never* restrain myself? When I saw that my pupils were unable to display their anger, *I* had to show them how it should be done. What a performance I gave! I had to outshine my class. Ah, yes! I had to do it brilliantly. I had to prove myself. I had to feel superior! *NITWIT!*

My own self-discoveries made me wonder why anybody chooses to work with the mentally ill. What motivates a person to select this particular field? The need to feel needed? The desire to control the uncontrollable? Is it the sensational aspect of psychotic behavior that is so fascinating? Do the patients serve *us* as objects of identification, of pity, of condescension? Do we need to project our own hang-ups onto the patients? Do we interpret their behavior from the viewpoint of our own conflicts? What had mine contributed to those botched sessions? I'll bet the outcome would have been very different if I'd been able to function without my hang-ups. I have to get rid of them. And I will!

I reviewed those sessions again and again. My three hours of mistakes as a dance therapist were becoming more and more valuable. What ·specific information had I picked up? Exactly what had I learned? I wrote down the results of my ponderings.

1. It is simply impossible to handle twenty-two patients in one class. Six or eight would be plenty, depending on each individual's tendency to cooperate.
2. Each group should consist of patients having more or less the same general disposition:
     Withdrawn patients
     Hyperactive patients
     Patients in fairly good contact
     Patients in poor contact
   After a while, there would be the possibility of combining them for purposes of variety and stimulation.
3. If one person's acting-out behavior—his need to "take over" any situation—disrupts the atmosphere of the class, I should take him out and work with him privately until his actions are modified by personal attention.
4. One-to-one sessions would also be necessary for patients out of contact.
5. Oh, and one more thing: the clothes the patients are

**Grouping patients**

36

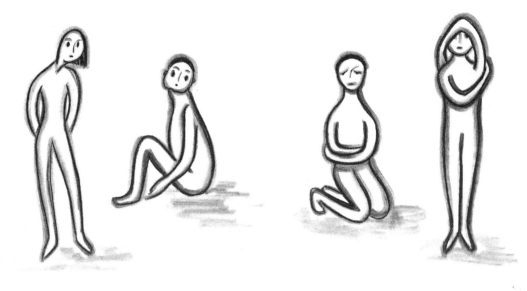

**Patients in fairly good contact**

**Patients in poor contact**

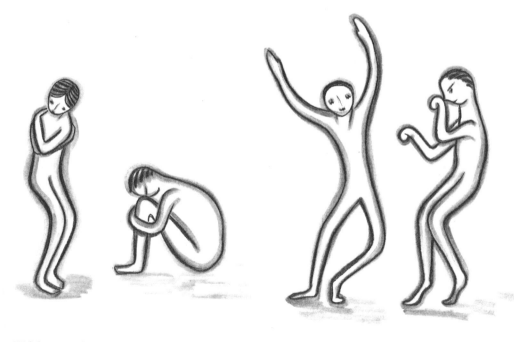

**Withdrawn patients**

**Hyperactive patients**

wearing—or *not* wearing—are just impossible. Suggest sweat suits for the men, leotards and wraparounds for the women. What a difference *that* would make!

Now then. Back to my own behavior. What had the patients taught me about myself?

1. *I must learn to be flexible.*

   I'd planned those sessions too carefully; so carefully that when the patients went off on a tangent, I panicked. I should accept such deviations as a positive indication of the personal expression I am seeking. A new theme could be developed from the patient's digression. My compliance wouldn't mean giving up my objective for that class; it would only represent a detour. If I had encouraged and supported them, if I had joined them in their wish for gymnastics, the patients would have felt that I approved of them and of their contribution. It could have been an active session if I'd grasped the opportunity to expand and vary their own movement theme. At the end, the strenuous exercises might have been readily exchanged for the quiet, swaying swings I'd wanted in the first place. Instead, I had kept myself apart: I had refused to join in on their level; had insisted on my own pre-planned ideas; and had given them no new movement experience. I had rejected their offering. *IDIOT!*

2. *I went too far, too fast.*

   "Invent a swing! What an unreasonable request *that* was! How would anyone know what a dancer means by a swing without first being taught its movement pattern, or shown its quality? And more of this nonsense: "Swing your bodies in any way you want!" Really! I was asking them to make a choice when they didn't even know what they were supposed to be making a choice *about!* They were helpless in the face of the freedom I so thoughtlessly demanded.

3. *Beware of imagery.*

   No one reacted to the images I gave to induce a swing.

Maybe they never saw wheatfields in the wind. Maybe they were afraid of ocean waves. Mightn't an image that seems harmless to me be threatening for them? I'd better go easy with this image-giving. Why not let the patients supply their own? I could ask them, "What does swinging remind you of?" Wouldn't that allow each patient to react out of his own experience? Wouldn't it encourage them to be actively involved, to be reliant on their own initiative instead of being passively dependent upon my suggestions? Besides, each person's image-association might give me valuable information about his nature. Who knows? He might even get information about himself!

4. *Emotions: Handle with care!*

When I asked my group to display anger, I was met by uncomprehending stares or by various acts of rebellion. Now I realize how naive I was in expecting a person to reveal his emotions, when for years he'd been preoccupied either in suppressing them or avoiding them. "I'm not angry, I never have *been* angry, and I never *will* be angry!" That flat statement should have been warning enough. But . . . I know that it's vitally important to bring those submerged feelings to the surface. The question is, HOW?

Well, I must face it: in every session, in every way, I demanded of the patients my way of feeling, my way of moving, my way of expressing myself. I behaved like a little dancing dictator—I, I, . . . Me, Me!

When I go back to the hospital, I'll really try to respond to the patient's needs. I'll go very slowly, as if I had a hundred years' time. I'll be open and flexible instead of insistent and domineering. I won't mute my pupils with my own exuberance, or shock them with my theatromania. I won't ask for creative movement before they have acquired a movement vocabulary to be creative with. Nor will I offer freedom until they can cope with it.

I started at the last paragraph I'd written. It began, "When

I go back to the hospital . . ." It seems that I've changed my mind. And saved myself a toll call.

One problem still remains unsolved: how can the patients' resistance to emotional expression be overcome? They had refused to acknowledge anger. The very word appeared to be threatening. How, then, can I ever bring their forbidden feelings out into the open without calling those feelings by name, without recourse to "the word"? I wonder. What if I use "the action" instead? I could apply the movements that are most commonly associated with a specific feeling—those that are universally recognized by anyone, anywhere on this earth. For example, if we see a person gasp sharply, widen his eyes, raise his shoulders, if the whole man suddenly tenses, contracts, aren't we witnessing sudden fear? Also, don't we know what a body is saying when its tension is light, its center lifted, when the feet skim the earth, the breathing is fluid, and the movements are open and free of contraction? Don't we express pleasure in this way? So, let's say I want to generate the feeling of anger. People stamp when they're mad, so I could use stamps. People punch; we could punch. People kick, slap, claw, pull, push. What would happen if a patient's body repeated such anger-forms, over and over? Would the anger-feeling erupt in spite of his need to conceal it? Could his body force him into the emotion? It's exciting to think about. . . .

Doesn't it seem strange, though, that I would separate action and feeling in order to restore a person's wholeness of being? Well, no, it isn't really so strange. Isn't anyone's state of mind constantly expressed by his body? And, vice versa, doesn't anyone's body-experience influence his state of mind? It doesn't seem to matter whether the process is initiated by the mind or by the body; the two conditions of being continue to interact and reinforce one another.

| Mental State | | Body Experience | Body Experience | | Mental State |
|---|---|---|---|---|---|
| Depression | causes | Slumping ←→ | Slumping | causes | Depression, etc. |
| Happiness | causes | Smiling ←→ | Smiling | causes | Happiness, etc. |
| Nervousness | causes | Twitching ←→ | Twitching | causes | Nervousness, etc. |
| Concentration | causes | Focusing ←→ | Focusing | causes | Concentration, etc. |

As for the patients, weren't their mental aberrations mirrored in their physical aberrations? And didn't their bodies' aberrations continue to reinforce the aberrations of their minds?

Of course, these illustrations are oversimplified. Any feeling can be expressed in a thousand different ways. But aren't the physical representations of a feeling based on identical *elements* of expression which occur reflexively in every one of us? Rhythmic patterns, positions, forms, movement designs, degrees of tension, use of space—these principles compose the mutual theme on which the individual performs his own variations. However unique a person's variations may be, we can all recognize the familiar elements that lie behind them. These elements provide the background for human understanding. They are universal; they apply to all people. They are the human expression!

But on the ward that first day I saw expressions that defied recognition. Normally, a person's expression changes with the advent of any new stimulus. His voice and movement acquire a different quality. His body projects a different feeling. So it was uncanny to see some of those patients communicate one and only one feeling, exhibit one and only one movement pattern, regardless of anything that went on around them. It was as if they had walled themselves off from any new experience.

Even more incomprehensible was the sight of two expressions permanently fixed in a single body. There was that man with the terribly sad face who sped so lightly about the ward. And the woman with the solidified smile who wanted to do battle with me—or anyone else within her reach. What happened to the interactive process here? Bodies don't skip when they're depressed. People don't hit when they're happy. Or do they?

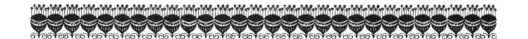

# SEPARATION AND UNITY
## Can't the Body Make Up Its Mind?

But wait now, haven't I discovered this two-way condition in my own body every so often? Sometimes, when I'm feeling perfectly content, with all signs of physical well-being, I realize that I've been pulling up my right shoulder until it aches from the strain. Why doesn't that shoulder agree with the rest of me? And how about Uncle Ulrich, talking in that tremendous, loud voice but never showing the same aggressiveness in his chest? It's all caved in, weak and soft looking. And what feeling is behind his right foot which taps and taps all the time? For once, can't his foot be quiet? Can't his voice be as soft as his chest? Can't his body make up its mind?

When I look at animals, what is it about their behavior, and what is it in their being that delights me so? When Blue, my golden retriever, runs after his ball, *all* of him runs. It's not only "Blue is running," it's "Running is Blue." And my beautiful cats, washing after dinner—that's categorical washing! Not one whisker has another idea.

Why do we humans find this oneness of being so difficult to come by? Even the best students in my regular dance classes frequently seem to be divided against themselves. In a turn, for instance, one body part will resist the whole idea of turning. A foot is left behind, the head stays put, a shoulder pulls back, as if debating the question: "To turn or not to turn?" And sometimes, though a person's physical structure may be dancing, his mind seems to be at home checking to find out if the gas is turned off, or thinking up brilliant rebuttals it could have made in last night's argument, or recalling mother's warning: "Be careful—you'll fall!" When you watch bodies dancing without cooperation from their minds, the lack of support becomes very obvious. The dance never becomes a full experience. To be sure, it's only human to let the mind ramble occasionally, but when signs of separation become constant, I begin to worry, and redouble my efforts to restore that person's unity.

I've gone on and on about the mind influencing the body. How about the body influencing the mind? Surely, we've all experienced the influence of our physical condition upon our mental state. If the body says it's cold, the mind thinks of sweaters. If the body complains of exhaustion, the mind orders rest. If the stomach says it's empty, the mind turns to thoughts of food. The trouble is that we don't always want to listen to what the body has to report. If we did listen, we humans wouldn't be such a nervous bunch, we wouldn't be so indecisive, we wouldn't be constantly overtired, we wouldn't be such an angry, confused generation. If our minds would only take the time to read the special delivery letters posted so urgently by our bodies.

CREDO

1. Man manifests himself in his body; the body is the visual representation of the total being.
2. Mind and body are in constant reciprocal interaction, so that whatever the inner self experiences comes to full realization in the body, and whatever the body experiences influences the inner self.
3. Whether thoughts and feelings are rational or irrational,

positive or negative, split or unified, acknowledged or inhibited, state of mind becomes embodied in the physical being. It is manifested in the body's alignment, in the way the body is centered, in its rhythmical patterns, in its tempo, sounds, use of tension and energy, in its relationship to space, in its potentiality for changes. All these factors determine the body's expression. They affect the way it moves, and moves about.

4. Through the body, man's mind experiences reality. His senses inform his mind of his very being. They tell him how he is, who he is, and where he is. Sight, sound, smell, taste, and touch incite his mental processes.

5. Mind and body are fused by their reciprocal interaction. Their collaboration insures human unity.

The mind-body partnership makes it possible for me to assume that a person can be influenced from either side of his nature. If psychoanalysis brings about a change in the mental attitude, there should be a corresponding physical change. If dance therapy brings about a change in the body's behavior, there should be a corresponding change in the mind. Both methods aim to change the total human, mind and body, which leads me to believe that if the psychotherapist and the dance therapist could be persuaded to join forces, the patient wouldn't stand a chance of maintaining his disturbance.

Because I've always been deeply involved with the expression of the body, and because my professional life has necessitated "reading" the body just as other people "study" the mind, it's only natural that I approach the area of mental disturbance from the viewpoint of the body's expression. I can only hope that the interactive process will justify my conviction that the body can influence even the desperately disturbed mind of the psychotic patient. The transformation of a patient's unfunctional physical distortions presents an enormous challenge, but I must try to reestablish for him a body that will again operate effectively and perform normally, a body that will have a positive, remedial effect upon his mind.

And what do I mean by a "normal" body? Precisely what do

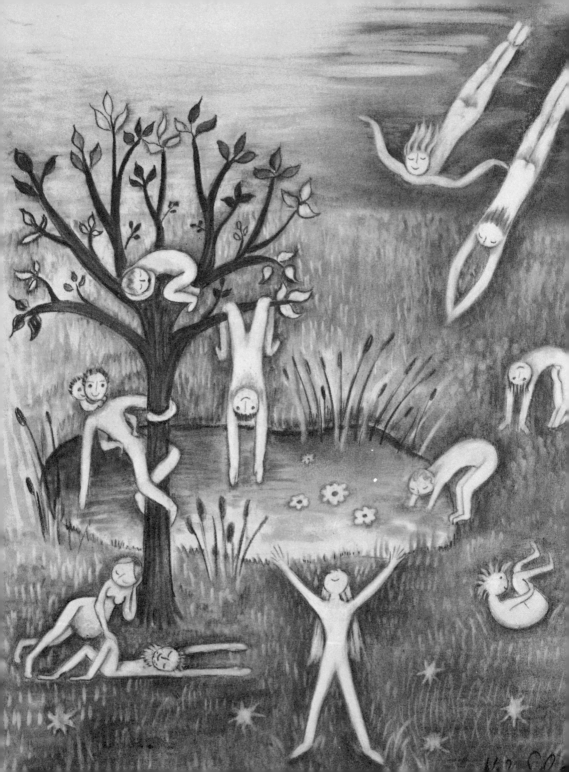

I think a body should be like after my dance "treatment"? How would it look, act, and feel? I'll certainly have to clarify my own concept of the body in its most ideal form. I'll need a "body-criterion" which can serve as a basis for comparative evaluation....

I envision a being, still in Paradise, living in joyous confirmation of itself, in accordance with its birth, its life, and its death, and proud of its ability to perpetuate its own image. It is a human form as it was meant to be and to function, in its complete, perfect state—revelling in its breathing, exulting in its motion, beautifully assertive in its total involvement with existence. It is an organic unity wherein mind and body are fused so that the thought is the action and the action is the thought. This being exists in the optimal center of gravity. It moves in balanced relationship between tension and release. Its breath adjusts and flows rhythmically. Its alignment is harmonious, well-centered, ready for change. Its muscle tone is functional, its movement and use of energy effective, and its adaptation to space spontaneous. Ever-curious, its senses are acutely tuned in to the sights, sounds, smells, tastes, and textures provided so lavishly by the environment. Delighting in all its possibilities, this body can make itself long or short, wide or narrow, big or small. It can walk, run, jump, leap, turn. It can kneel, crouch, sit, lie down. It can stand on two feet, on one foot—or on its head. It falls, climbs, swims. All such doings can reflect any quality—strong or soft, heavy or light, active or passive—and be pleasurably performed in any tempo, from the slowest to the fastest. And the whole marvelous conglomeration can be limitlessly changed, rearranged, organized to suit any human desire, anywhere, at any time.

Such a body wholeheartedly transforms its feelings into appropriate physical manifestations. It shouts in joy, hisses in anger, laughs in amusement, strikes out in hatred, blushes in shame, sobs in grief, relaxes in contentment. It contracts in pain, slumps in exhaustion, stutters in excitement, blocks in fear, yields in love, splits in indecision, and disintegrates in confusion. Constantly and adequately, this body performs its feelings.

Whenever an emotional reaction has been expressed, the ideal body regains its equilibrium. It returns to its point of departure, its home base, which provides the full, unrestricted potential for new experience. Here, any contraction, distortion, or cramp can be released into the most capable, effortless, enjoyable body-feeling. Here, the body will become well grounded if it has flown too high, fluid if it has been blocked, reassembled if it has fallen apart, revitalized if its energy has been exhausted. Like a pendulum, this being can swing back and forth between reaction and resolution. Within this stabilizing process, emotion has been given full physical expression; the ideal being has embodied its feeling. Whatever the affective experience, it has taken its course, has been given a form, has been changed, has been resolved. No residue remains to color future encounters. . . . Such was the perfect body I envisioned.

But as I looked closely at my own body and at the bodies of my fellow men, I realized how very, very little they had to do with paradise. Where had all the beauty gone—the lust for change, the spontaneity, the happy involvement? Where had we hidden our feelings? In which closet had we stored away our tenderness? Where had we buried our aggression? Why were we so pitifully inactive? Why so miserably inhibited? What became of the one-ness, the harmonious unity? The people on the street or on the farms or in the offices—the girl next door, the housewife, the "big shots," the average man—thee and me: whatever happened to us?

Are there basic similarities between the disturbances in our bodies and the enormous distortions in the bodies hidden behind the walls of mental hospitals? Can the two be equated in any way? Is it a matter of degree? Or is there a definite line of distinction—visible, tangible, understandable? Perhaps a long, hard look at man in my time, within my own range of association, can open the door to a deeper comprehension.

**From wherever we came**

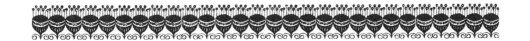

# THE UNFORTUNATE LEGACY

## *"You Ought to be Ashamed of Yourself!"*

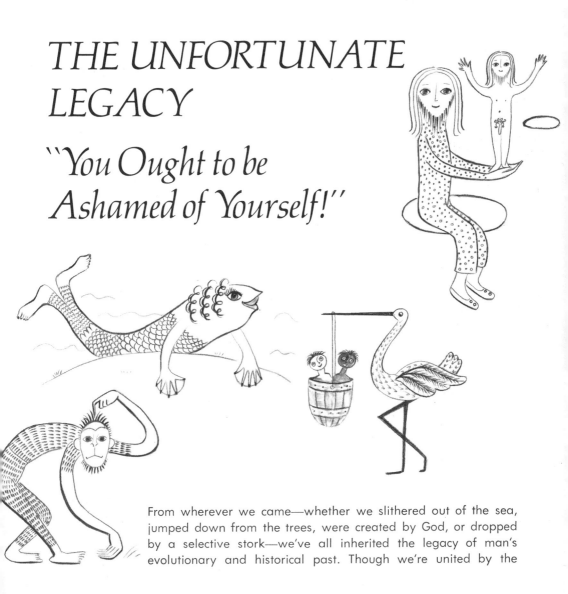

From wherever we came—whether we slithered out of the sea, jumped down from the trees, were created by God, or dropped by a selective stork—we've all inherited the legacy of man's evolutionary and historical past. Though we're united by the

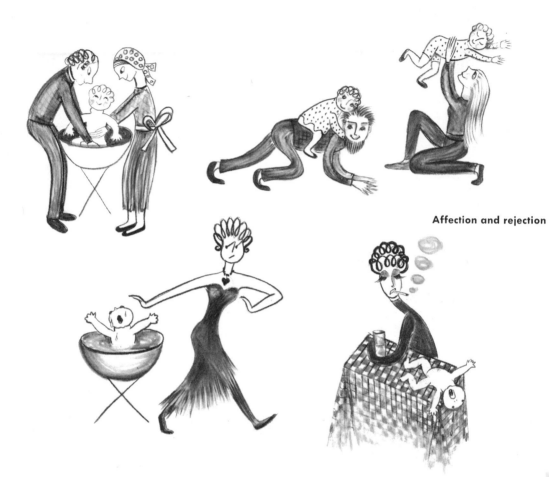

basic blueprint of our physical structure, the species "man" some-how manages to come in an enchanting assortment of colors, shapes, sizes, intellects, feelings, and behaviors. All the varied aspects of heredity and all the diversified possibilities of environ-ment combine with each person's essential nature to form a unique being. How fascinating to realize that any body enters this earth with the possibility of becoming a very special Somebody!

But so much seems to depend upon the way any human is received into this world. Does the brand new body feel welcome, loved? Does it feel lost, rejected? The emotional climate envelop-ing earliest infancy seems to lay the foundation of a human's

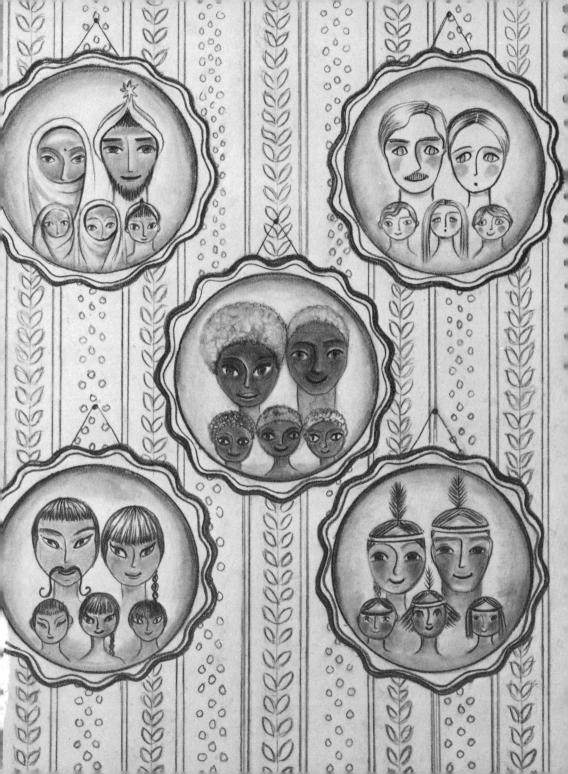

self-image. If his vulnerable form is cared for with warmth and respect and affection, he stands a good chance to be on good terms with it for the rest of his life, and will be able to appreciate himself and give love and trust to others. If it is treated coldly or callously, the stage is set for future self-dislike and physical incompatibility. From infancy onward, the incipient "Somebody" is bombarded by formative influences—within the family structure and outside of it—that can either damage or encourage his opinion of himself.

This body of ours has such tremendous potential for giving and receiving pleasure. It seems tragic that all through the ages, the reigning moral codes have brandished it threateningly over our heads, declaring it "sinful," "dirty," "evil," "dangerous," and something unsavory that must be covered up. The natural appreciation for our physical being has often been denied us. But if we can't love our own bodies, how can we possibly love the bodies of others?

The inhibiting of the body begins very early in life. As soon as possible—or sooner—children are carefully taught what their anatomy is allowed and *not* allowed to do. "Don't be such a cry-baby!" "Quit that silly giggling!" "Sit still and be quiet!" "If you don't stop playing with yourself, I'll tie up your hands!" "Get down out of that tree before you break your neck!" "Don't touch me—you're a mess!" "Stop asking so many ridiculous questions!" And the ultimate squelch: "You ought to be ASHAMED OF YOURSELF!" As a child tries desperately to conform, he begins to censor his feelings, contain his curiosity, limit his action, and suppress any behavior that is contradictory to the desired image being thrust upon him by the older people—the "Ones Who Know." Lesson learned: *Spontaneity is taboo.*

Of course, every human is part of some sort of society which enables its members to function together. If we want to benefit from the society, we must live within its dictates. That would be work enough for the individual if it ended there. But along with the lawful behavior that any society prescribes, there is also a "social behavior" demanded of us which often seems totally irrelevant to our relationship to the rest of the group. Why must the personal habits that are socially acceptable be so artificial? Why

**Tortures of fashi**

do we have to quirk our little fingers when handling a teacup? Why are elbows so outmoded? Why is bent-kneed slouching so gorgeous? And lily-white hands so desirable? Why is the affected whisper so appealing? Why do we confuse boredom with grace? Why do we connect polished behavior with a minimum of movement? It seems to be an established fact that the less we show of ourselves, the more we are considered to be charming and elegant.

Must we also find it necessary to suppress, alter, or deny our physical expression in order to be good citizens? Must we disguise our emotions, masking a very real sorrow with a determined smile, or a beautiful exhilaration with a bland, composed visage? If only we were at liberty to show how we honestly feel! If only our bodies didn't have to lie, and pretend, and behave so falsely! If only we could be free to enjoy ourselves as we really are!

Not only is the body told how it should behave, it is also given instructions about how it should look. And the "in-look" changes with distracting frequency. Dissatisfaction with our physical image has been intriguingly illustrated by the way we have altered the body's appearance. All through the centuries, we've managed to invent an amazing variety of fashionable devices

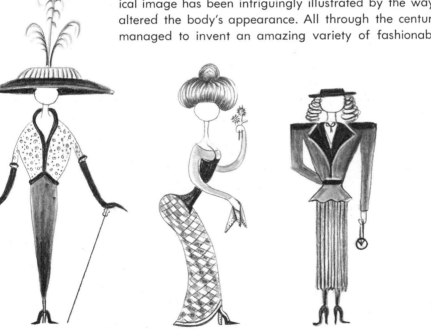

with which to hide, camouflage, exaggerate, or idolize various parts of the human form. We have a positive genius for constructing paddings, wire contraptions, bonings, corsettings, elaborate trimmings and trappings—all to either minimize or maximize our natural contours. During the course of history, women's waistlines have wandered up and down the body. Bosoms have contracted or expanded. Rumps have bulged alarmingly or been squashed flat. Flesh has been exposed or hidden, added to or subtracted from. Faces have been remodelled with paint and pencil and the surgeon's skill. Feet have been propped up on spike heels. Throats have been choked by constricting collars. Yes, fashion has always declared the *en vogue* state of our bodies' appearance. But isn't it strange that man's deep-rooted urge to play with forms and color have so often resulted in such discomfort for his body? And don't fashion's hectic fluctuations sometimes seem a little bit puzzling? Shoulder-length hair, once the crowning glory of our beloved saints, is now looked upon by many with disgust. And isn't it bewildering that the beard, which not too long ago represented a man of consequence, a solid citizen, has in a scant few years generally become the maligned and detested symbol of all that is wrong with the younger generation?

Man's mind has certainly been exercising itself since time on earth began. Its spectacular scientific achievements have radically changed the environment. Its brilliant technological discoveries have served us well. Too well. Designed specifically for our comfort and protection, they have bedded man's body soft and safe. It lies quite dormant. Normally, a present-day human doesn't have to fight for his life, climb for his safety, run to a hiding-place, attack an enemy. No, the bodies of our best young men must be precisely trained in such lost skills so that they can go out and do battle for us. We can rest secure in our cosy quiescence. Especially in the Western world, planes and cars do our running for us; machines labor for us; furnaces and air-conditioners temper our climate; processing plants prepare more and more so-called food for us; water spouts from a billion faucets; night becomes day or day becomes night at the flick of a switch. In the process of adjusting to the mechanized world, our bodies began to lie fallow. There has simply been no necessity for physical exertion. Man has succeeded, after centuries of intellectual toil, in liquidating the agility and self-sufficiency of his entire organism.

Since man no longer needs to fight physically for his existence, his natural aggression has been dangerously suppressed. But the drive still remains within each one of us. Denied any outlet, it can build to an intolerable intensity that may erupt in wildly irrational acts of violence. The assailant seems always to be the sort of person who "never caused a moment's worry to his parents," a hard-working, straight-A student, a Boy Scout leader, a clean-living churchgoer, who suddenly picks up a rifle and begins slaughtering his fellowman. Once vital for survival, aggression has lost its original reason to be. We are still in tragic confusion as we seek a direction for this powerful drive.

None of us escapes the conditioning of heredity, of environment and social structure, or of changes wrought by mankind in time. Despite the limitless differentiations of our encounters, there is one experience we all share in common. Every human has faced, is facing, will always have to face his confrontation with death. Most significant is the way we face it. Man certainly knows, deep down, that sooner or later his body will cease to exist—at least in its present form—but he is not so sure how his spirit will behave.

How does he cope with the obscurity of his destiny? Does he coddle or fortify his body in a dedicated effort to preserve it? Does he, in advance, try to become detached from his troublesome dilemma of a body and prepare his soul for an everlasting journey through eternity? Does he gamble with death, betting his life on his body's permanence? Does he hasten his body's demise in anticipation of a final resting place? Man's attitude toward these questions fundamentally affects the way he treats his body.

If a person is supremely confident of a "life hereafter," his body can become a welcome mat for death. Intellectual and spiritual pursuits take precedence over his physical being, which is merely a necessary housing for mind and soul. As such, it requires a minimum of attention. Its immediate needs, desires,

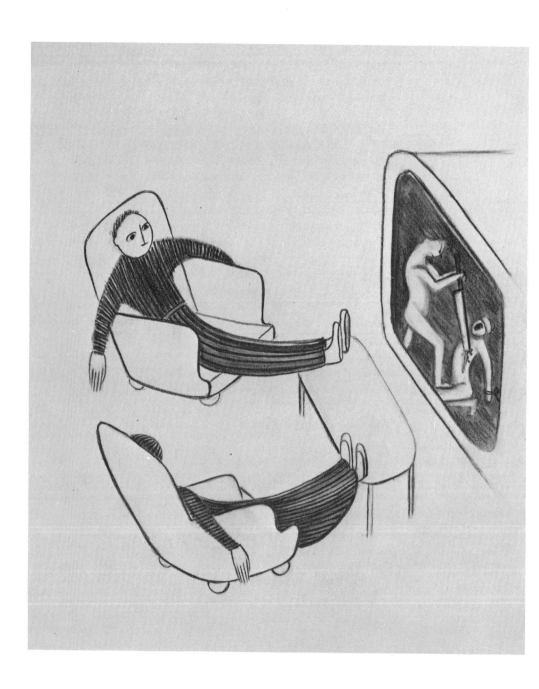

and functions can be neglected to the extent that it loses its talent for living.

What if a person can't accept the comfortable possibility of an enduring soul, and dreads the extinction of his being? Then the wish that his body might live forever becomes the essence of his life. He does everything he can to preserve it. In abject fear, he listens to his heartbeat, feels his pulse, takes his temperature, watches his body's functions. He seems to feel that if, so far, his body has made it, any change could only be for the worse. This fragile structure, never exposed or energized, is degraded to a state of hibernation—a lifeless form which, hopefully, death may overlook.

Another man may take the active role in the preservation of his physical self. Ignoring his mind, he attempts to develop a superbody, a monster of resistance, which death cannot conquer. Strict and stern, he trains his heart for endurance, his lungs for volume, his muscles for strength, his legs for running, his arms for lifting. Bulging and straining, this colossal muscle-bundle applies his own strenuous formula for longevity.

Sometimes, death is felt to be the final punishment after being sentenced to life. We behave toward it in the same way that a guilt-ridden child deliberately provokes the chastisement of an angry parent. To this category of "death-challengers" belong the adventurers, auto-racers, aerialists, wild-animal hunters, glacier-scalers. See how mankind "plays with fire," marches up to the cannon's mouth," "sleeps on volcanos." How exciting to feel oneself so much alive! Isn't Russian roulette fun?

In its ultimate form, the urge to detach from the physical being leads a person to rid himself completely of this symbol of fear. He may strike out at the bodies of his fellowmen, murdering individually or en masse, or destroy his own body in the final horror of suicide.

**Spectators of life** Whatever method man uses to escape the fact of the body's transience, he necessarily becomes immune to feelings. The less we feel our bodies, the less we lose when they disintegrate. The less we enjoy our bodies, the easier it is to part from them. *The less we live, the less we die.* Thus, the fear of death becomes the fear of life.

So here we are, spectators of life, condemned to a state of placid passivity, experiencing life's diversity only vicariously. Instead of living our own lives, we try to live with an illustration of life that others perform for us, thereby replacing sensory involvement with intellectual observation. See the housewives weeping empathic tears with the heroine of the daily soap opera. See the sports fans, provided with the opportunity to feed on vitality and agility when, in abstraction, they run with the track men. During an evening of theatrical drama we can live the life of the hero or the villain, admiring the aggression and drives that the actors express and that we, ourselves, suppress. Gazing upon the spot-lit glamour of a ballet, we can identify with the "ideal" bodies of the dancers, the beautifully functional movements which are now lost to us. Parked in plush comfort, we can watch others do our suffering, loving, hating, destroying, crying, laughing, living, and dying for us. Like graven images we sit, and sit, and sit, and the degree of our involvement—if it comes high—can only be shown in the amount and volume of our applause.

Perhaps my "perceptions of mankind viewed collectively" seem to be exaggerated, my illustrations oversimplified. I only know that I hardly ever see a body openly and adequately portray an emotion; physical expression is too often altered, suppressed, or denied altogether. Rarely does a body seem to be respected, appreciated, enjoyed. At best, it is clean but colorless. At worst, it has become an object of shame and fear. Gone is the capacity for effective action. Lost is the freedom to communicate thoughts and feelings. The body's vital partnership with the mind is on very shaky grounds. All in all, we've managed to disregard our bodies' natural birthright.

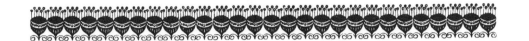

# THE SILENT MESSAGE
## The Body is a Blabbermouth

Thrust into the vortex of universal human experience, the individual is simultaneously subjected to the influence of his own specific world. The variety of his distinctively personal encounters and confrontations, the vast array of his particular choices and decisions, the singularity of his actions and reactions, make man what he is—alone and unique in a communal existence.

How inconceivable it is, considering the billions of people in this world, that no two are identical, certainly not in looks, and definitely not in actions. Watch people walking, standing, sitting. Watch people shopping, talking, waiting. Watch people smoking, eating, reading. See how humans cry, laugh, love, reject, accept. See them being shocked, scared, curious, greedy, jealous. Careful scrutiny will show that every man, woman, and child has his own distinctive feeling reaction to any one experience. If a group of people is confronted by a singular emotion-provoking situation, not one person in that group will have the

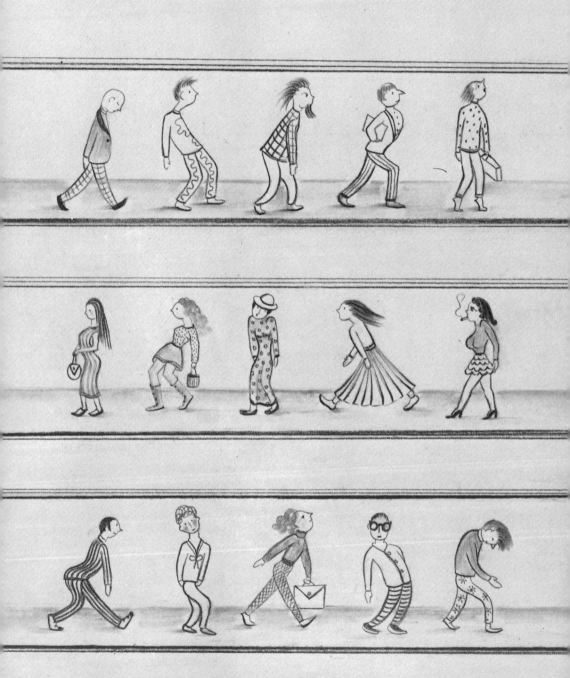

exact same body response. In fear, one may run away, another collapse, while a third attacks. An angry man may scowl, bare his teeth, roll his eyes—or smile. He may tease, strike out, or sulk. Depressed people may show their desolation by unfocussed staring, by motionless silence, or by ceaseless talking. Their bodies may droop or stiffen up. One person may mourn at home, while another may rush out to buy new clothes. A happy mood can be revealed in tears or in laughter, in sharing or in secrecy, in excited movement or in quietude. There's no doubt that the "specialty" of each individual is vividly shown in the expression of his body.

It seems to me that each body I see radiates its own non-verbal message, and that this message represents the sum total of the individual's various characteristics. By means of its un-spoken projection, I can sense a personality as being funda-mentally open or closed, active or passive, aggressive or defensive. I can see reflections of protest, compliance, acceptance, rejection, affirmation, confirmation, or secrecy. It may convey a strong sense of self or a lack of self-respect. But again, I feel that the most significant of all body-statements is the one that indicates a person's feeling about his own body. He may love it, hate it, or take it for granted. But whatever his prevailing attitude, it will surely influence his relationship to the world around him.

Consciously or unconsciously, we all respond to the mute self-declarations of our fellowmen. We may react with interest, rejection, or apathy. We may experience a distinct sensation of uneasiness about a person before he has opened his mouth. We may accept the notion of "love at first sight" or of "instant dis-like." We may have a sense of such complete familiarity with a total stranger that it seems we've known him forever.

**Watch people walking**

Every one of us has been on the receiving end of "good vibes" and "bad vibes." Don't we all know the individual who radiates a warmth that can light up the darkest atmosphere? And the somebody among us whose air of gloomy foreboding silences any laughter, freezes any motion? Then there's the family at their dinner table: hanging over the meal, like an omnipresent chandelier, is the particular family's atmosphere. It may be for-mal and oppressive, friendly and relaxed, or stern and inflexible.

61

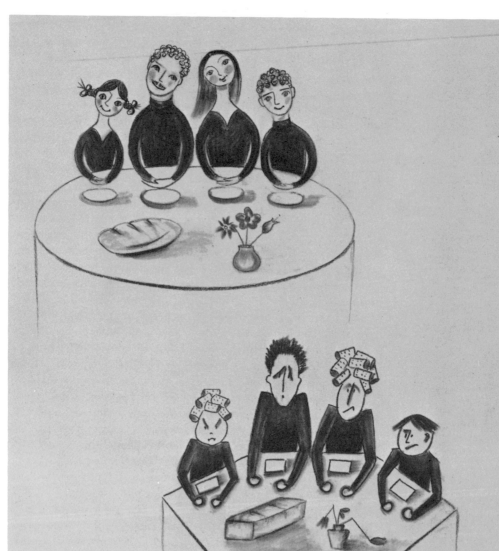

The food may be consumed with anxiety and indigestion, with joy and camaraderie, or in isolation and silence. Does Mother set the mood as well as the table? Or does Father clamp it down as he descends into his chair? Whoever decrees the "family-feeling-at-dinner-time," there is no doubt about its contagious effect on all assembled. Why do we react so readily to the vibrations of another person? Surely not by means of any kind of black magic. No, we are responding simply and directly to the individual's body expression.

The body broadcasts our conflicts as well as our moods. How often we stand at a crossroad in our feelings, torn between duty and pleasure, love and hate, should and should not, right and wrong, going or staying. We verbalize our problematic situations quite explicitly: "I'm on the fence." "My feelings are divided." "I'm of two minds on the subject." "I'm really torn." Now let's see how people's bodies act out their temporary conflicts.

Watch a small boy, joyously involved in a ball game with his gang, when his mother calls him home "right now!" Stock still he stands, instantly immobilized by the conflict between duty and pleasure. Then a despairing groan accompanies his body's thawing-out process. Grudgingly, the boy wends his way across the yard with all the alacrity of a snail. Leaden legs drag along the rest of his body, which is wrenched into the opposite direction in a futile effort to stay in the game. He's split in two . . . until he hears, "Hurry up, your steak's getting cold!" Instantly, he's off at a dead run for the house, his whole body zipping like an arrow through space, every body part in full agreement with his stomach and the "duty"!

We are all only too familiar with that devastating moment when everything happens at once. A prime example is the housewife who has just answered the telephone, when, as if on cue, the children start a screaming fight, the Fuller Brush man rings the doorbell, and the coffee boils over on the stove. Friendliness, fury, anxiety, and desperation collide in physical sync: face frozen in a witless grin, left hand clutching the phone, right arm brandishing wildly at the kids, one leg caught in a giant step toward the door on the right, the other in a giant step toward the kitchen on the left, the whole disassembled body transfixed in

**Families at the dinner table**

its disintegration—as the fuse blows! Let's just leave her there in the dark. We know she'll settle it somehow. She always does.

The end-of-the-party conflict starts when all the guests simultaneously realize it's 3 A.M. In a concerted effort to end the evening, everyone jumps up at once. There's a race to open the front door . . . and there they remain. Deadlocked. In the freezing cold. The battle between going and staying begins. Their weights shift from side to side. Their feet dance a nervous pro and con. With the slightest move to go, the chatter increases in volume, the gestures in range and tempo, and the smiles in width. Each time the departure miscarries, the entire action is reversed. Back and forth the bodies pendulate, like tired metronomes.

Frequently, two feelings of equal intensity simultaneously invade the body. Accordingly, it projects an ambiguous, two-way image. A frowning-smiling face, a composed-nervous body accepting-rejecting movements, a tremulous-aggressive voice are only a few physical indications that separate feelings are temporarily coexisting within the same body.

Consider a wedding reception. The closest family friend embraces the bride with sincere tenderness, then easily moves about, conversing pleasantly with the guests, her whole smiling attitude a warm contribution to the happiness of the people she loves. But, almost invisibly, one clenched fist beats a furious staccato close to her side. It signals anger, still being experienced after an unresolved argument with her husband. Love and rage compete for her body's expression.

The permissive mother finally *must* punish her beloved child. As adoration conflicts with severity, see her sorrowful face, hear her apologetic voice, as they resist the decisive disciplinary action taken by her hands—is it a slap or a love-pat?

A person may consciously try very hard to conceal one of his two coexisting emotions. But the body, in its preoccupation with honesty, somehow manages to smuggle in the truth. The next time you have friends over for a poker game, peek under the table at the lower halves of those card-playing bodies. Watch the restlessly tapping feet, the legs twining around each other like grapevines, the knees either plastered together or jouncing up and down. Then take a look at the upper halves of those bodies *above* the table. Behold the easy, relaxed postures, the serenely confident gestures, the bland poker faces.

Did you ever see a man being told off by an unreasonable boss? Didn't the iron tension in his clamped jaw belie his subservient posture, his apologetic gestures? You'll find that clues to a two-way feeling are fairly easy to detect in any body. But when there are three, or four, or more feelings in combat, it's almost impossible to isolate the individual expressions.

Having to deal with conflicting feelings can be a wearing process. So much so, that some of us seem to avoid utilizing the wide variety of emotions at our disposal. It's as if such a person finds it more comfortable to settle for a single attitude, which at one particular time in life may have served a special purpose or filled an essential need. He seeks to conceal other facets of his nature which would interfere with the one image he's chosen to exhibit to the world.

This oversimplified being can be spotted anywhere, but his behavior is especially remarkable when he feels exposed. At any social gathering, the "Life of the Party" bounces into the room with explosive greetings and uproarious laughter, boisterously grabbing, shaking, and back-slapping everyone in sight with loving violence. The "Loner" sits isolated in a corner, separate and remote, his body maintaining its needed distance. Then there is the "Martyr": the door opens and in comes a man offering his chest to be stabbed, his hand to be cut off, his back to be beaten, his face to be slapped, bravely inviting the annihilation of his whole self. Surely we've all met the "Living Apology," the "People-Pleaser," the "Snob," the "Burden-Bearer," the "Wet Blanket," the "Heel," and the "Do-Gooder." The procession of one-sided characters goes on and on.

However a person typecasts himself, it's amazing to see how his body leaps to the fore with its gift for unmistakable characterization. It mobilizes every functioning element to reinforce the required attitude. If the image of "Power" is to be projected, the body becomes a solid block, with every joint rigid, inflexible. Perpetually upright and towering it stands, feet apart and firmly rooted to the earth. The center is clutched in its own iron grip, exercising unyielding control over the entire body. Each muscle is tensed and ready, the shoulders braced for bearing sudden weights, the chest fully expanded. Breathing is slow and measured, as are words, as are any necessary movements. There stands a marble monument of a man.

And what about the body that only conveys shyness? The quivering center opens a little, then retreats a lot, drawing the feeble extremities along with it. Every muscle in the entire structure follows this pattern of vacillation between opening and closing—with emphasis on the closing. The shallow breathing catches and releases in the same irregular pattern. The eyes peek out but quickly look down again. The voice begins a sentence, but swallows the end of it. The face alternately flushes and pales while the feet shift back and forth. The helpless hands hover up and down the front of the body, trying to hide various vulnerable parts. Every physical possibility reinforces the expression of shame.

Not only as individuals do we enact descriptive parts in the drama of life. Practically every group within our society seems to adopt a uniform physical front which projects the role the individuals have united to play. Easily recognizable is the distinguished elegance of the Beautiful People, the colorful sloppiness of the hippies, the corsetted authority of the military, the "busy-bodies" of dedicated clubwomen, the hate personification of revolutionaries. And any group attitude can be further simplified and abstracted by a symbolic gesture: the raised fist of the black militant, the grim thrust of the Hitler salute, the reverent obeisance of the sign of the cross, the two-fingered peace sign. But whatever the one-sided feeling representation may be, and however it is displayed, I'm sure that even the most determined role-player battles in private with all the human conflicts that he publicly ignores.

Most of us can, and do, find solutions to life's continuous barrage of transitory conflicts. The indeterminate situation may resolve itself, but ideally we make our own decisions, draw our own conclusions, clarify our own emotional positions. We establish a point of view which enables us to assume responsibility for whatever action we've finally chosen to take. Once a decision has been reached, we can cease the passive wavering between two positions. Usually, the moment a conflict has been resolved,

**Symbolic gestures**

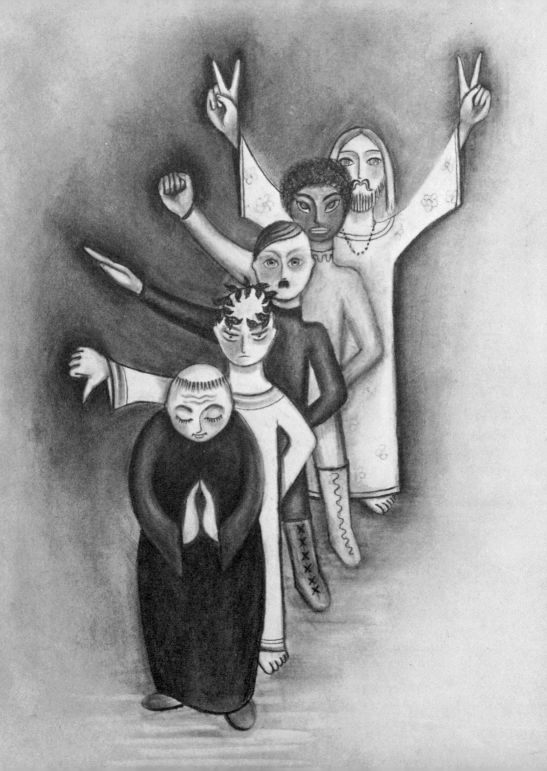

we instinctively regain our functional equilibrium, with no remaining physical token to interfere with our body's free performance.

However, the pros and cons of a particular decision can remain with a person for years. An identical stressful situation may be relentlessly reinforced; a pair of contrasting emotions may persist for a lifetime. Whatever the cause, this body continues to display the chronic problem. No matter how well-adjusted we are, I believe that every one of us is stamped to a certain degree by unresolved conflicts, either in the whole body or in at least one body part. The entire body may lean slightly backward, as if in permanent avoidance. It may slant forward, in an attitude of constant challenge. The whole physical unit may surrender to the force of gravity with a continually dragged-down appearance, or it may resist contact with the earth, stretching ever skyward. It may dawdle deliberately or race riotously down the road of life. In the body's isolated parts, we may see hunched shoulders or out-thrust chests or tilted heads or arched spines or clenched fists or retracted pelvises or locked knees or . . . or . . . or . . . . Feet may drag or bounce, walk on eggs or on clouds, or slog through mud. There are the cross-legged knee-bouncers, the toe-and-finger-tappers, the hair-pullers, the scratchers, and the rubbers, and the twitchers, and the yellers, and the whisperers.

Needless to say, any habitual representation of a conflict inhibits the body's functional action. It isn't easy to run if we lean backward. It's pretty hard to make love with a retracted pelvis. With a cramped, stiff body we can't very well put up a good fight, do our work adequately, or converse effectually with a friend. We can't give with closed hands, or caress with a fist. We can't talk, call, or sing with a tight, closed throat. It's impossible to rest if we twitch, rub, or scratch.

Disturbed feelings which are so fixed in the body not only reduce and inhibit the physical ability for free performance; they also color any new encounter with life. All future experiences will be influenced by whatever feeling originally created the body's deviation from the functional norm. With pulled-up shoulders, we respond to any situation by whatever these pulled-up shoulders represent. With tightly crossed arms, we experience life "tightly crossed." We are prevented from experiencing spontaneously and realistically. Our expectation is fixed.

We have so many ways to inhibit, camouflage, underplay, overstate, and misrepresent our feelings that it isn't always easy to read any person's physical message. But as a movement therapist, I can see the problem in the body and must try my best to resolve that problem by changing its visible symbol.

Such are my reflections upon the bodies of "ordinary" people as they exist in my time and society—anchored in the past, apprehensive of the future, wasteful of the present. How sharply this picture contrasts with my image of the ideal form and its ability to resolve the negative experiences of the past, so that these experiences cannot burden the anticipation of the future or interfere with active involvement in the present.

Thus far, we've only looked at the bodies of people who function somehow . . . live anyhow . . . some for better, many for worse. But they are the fortunate beings we call "sane." What, then, of the others? Our society calls a human "normal" if he can adjust to its laws and demands, if he feels and behaves basically like the majority. But from time to time, a person may create his very own world, with its own precepts, and inhabitants. This person has his own time and space, his own customs, manners, and sensations. He has no interest in what we call "reality," and we other earthlings cannot enter his fantastic kingdom. Considering all such deviations from our norm, we determine that a person is lost in a world manufactured by his emotional disturbance.

We have had no other recourse, up to now, except to separate him from the rest of society. He has become a threat to us and to himself. Within his place of seclusion, we hope to teach him that the reality he has fled can be dealt with, can be challenged, can even be a pleasure. And as we try to coax him back to us, we call him "patient." How I dislike this label! To me, he is less a "mental case" and much more a fascinating foreigner. This attitude prevents me from regarding him as "sick." It merely assumes that he is different, exotic. We may have difficulties understanding each other, but I am determined to learn his

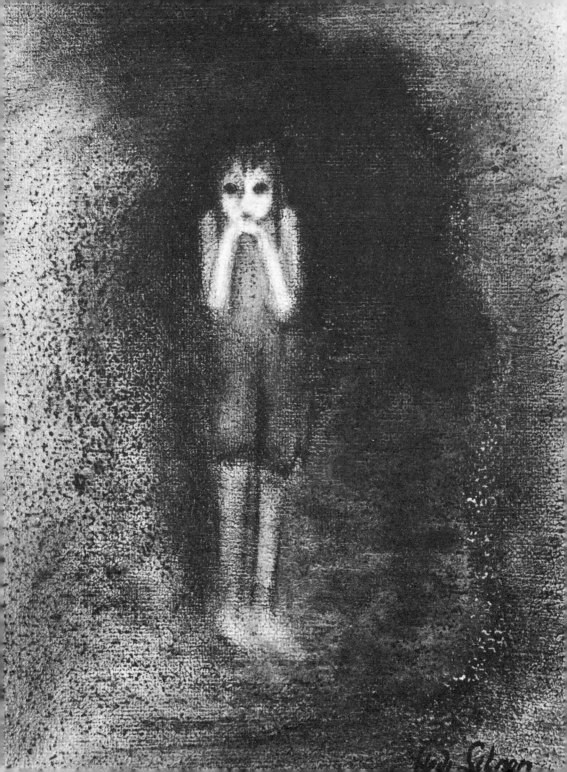

language, his customs, and I would give anything to know who rules his country. As long as I feel this way, I have no need to fear him, pity him, or condescend to him. I can only treat our "aliens" with full deference for their uniqueness. Whoever they are, it is to these special persons that this discussion is dedicated —with my love and respect.

**It is to these people . . .**

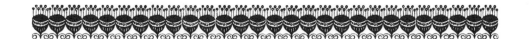

# THE PRIMACY OF PLEASURE

## Creeping Toward Dance

### Mary

A weird phenomenon is created by the relentless repetition of the psychotic's bizarre body attitudes and movements. To gain trust and establish initial contact, I try to experience those strange physical manifestations myself. I ally my body with the bodies of the patients. If I do what they do, somehow I feel how they feel. And one day, the understanding will be mutual.

Mary was one of my first "private pupils." She was a young black woman with a healthy-looking body, tall and erect. For three years—as long as she'd been in the hospital—no one had ever heard her speak. She didn't have to . . . the expression on her strong face let everyone around her know in no uncertain terms that she was furious. Mary's eternal, restless pacing gave the impression that she was angrily but methodically measuring the forty-foot distance between the walls. As she strode back and forth, in unvarying rhythm and stride, I moved along beside her, trying to match both her mood and her action. Our irate partnership must have presented an odd picture; Mary's very long legs covered ground so swiftly that I had to sprint in order to keep up with her.

After a couple of weeks, I made a small change in the pattern. I began to stretch out one friendly hand toward my companion's clenched fist. Then, for months, I did nothing else every day for half an hour but trot along at her side, offering my hand to her. All this while, she treated me like air, never uttering a sound, never giving any indication that she knew I existed. Then one day, in the midst of our lonely *pas de deux*, Mary did it! Her arm shot out and she grasped my hand. Just as abruptly, she flung it away. But from this split second of fleeting contact, Mary began her long struggle to relinquish her isolation. One day she would seem a little friendlier. Another day she looked angry again. Sometimes she would hold my hand for quite a while, then not take it again for a week. During all this time, she had never once looked at me. But at last there came the day when her gaze met mine. Those inward-seeing eyes had become focused and direct. Not only was I sure that she recognized my presence, but it also seemed that she had begun to like the person who shared her need for pacing. It is a profoundly touching experience: to be included at last in another person's world after working in a vacuum for so many months, to be given the right to intrude upon such monumental privacy.

On the basis of her tacit permission, I could now go ahead and gradually widen the range of Mary's compulsive behavior. We played all sorts of "pacing games": who could pace in different directions, who could pace with an open mouth, with bent knees, with crossed fingers, who could pace the slowest, who could stand still between paces, who could sit or lie down the longest, and, finally, who could not want to pace anymore.

One morning, after an exhausting session of pacing jumps and hopping paces, we both sank wearily to the floor and sat there, staring at each other. I was feeling frustrated. After eight months of almost daily companionship, I had never heard one word from my silent partner. I was still talking into a void. It seemed that I couldn't stand the omnipresent stillness one more minute.

"You know, Mary," I said, "I really feel terribly lonesome!"

Her great brown eyes widened with astonishment. Miraculously, the long-buried voice came forth to meet me.

"You feel lonesome, Trudi??"

Gooseflesh pricked my arms. My spine froze. The shock was so electrifying that for a moment, *I* could not speak. I reached over and gave her a hug.

"It's okay, Mary. I'll see you tomorrow."

"Right, Trudi!" And Mary smiled.

The long months of our seclusive partnership had been rewarded. Generally freed of her movement pattern as well as her self-imposed silence, Mary could now be admitted into one of my classes.

It isn't likely that Mary's breakthrough could ever have occurred publicly, in a group situation. Most severely withdrawn patients seem to need a confidant, one person with whom they can finally share their secrets, their hidden conflicts. It's also necessary to work alone with an individual whose "acting-out" conduct will reduce a group session to a shambles. Any acute behavior manifestation can be more easily coped with in private. Alone with a person, I can give him the full support and attention he so desperately needs. What's more, he doesn't have to defend himself against so many. His adversaries are reduced to one! But occasionally the one-to-one encounter proves to be too threatening. A patient may feel uncomfortably exposed when he's the sole focal point of observation. My personal feeling is that the atmosphere of a private session can sometimes become too serious and clinical. The patient brings with him only his singular, all-pervasive mood, which can so easily set the climate that it is more difficult for me to realize my objective goal.

Of course, I truly *enjoy* working with a group. Very rarely are all the patients gloomy, or apathetic, or exhilarated at the same time, so the different feeling representations constantly stimulate my working ideas. And for the patient, the group is invaluable. It permits him to grow at his own pace. He doesn't have to react immediately, respond personally, to suggestions which are made to the whole class. He can postpone the effort to change until he is ready. Also, the group represents a realistic life situation. Its members are pulled together into a unit as they interact with the therapist. They seem to develop a feeling of belonging, like a family that has been thrown into the same destiny, for better or for worse. Very quickly, they form a sense of responsibility toward one another. Though I work with very violent men and women from time to time, I seldom have to worry. The patients themselves usually take care of any intimidating situation that might arise. And as the children in a family share a parent, the group members must share the therapist. The attachment which necessarily occurs never seems to become too desperate. What's more, the class structure gives me the opportunity to bring the whole furtive secrecy about the body out into the open. The body's intimacy is shared with others in a most pleasant and natural way.

Above all, the group allows me to create a climate of child-like playfulness and humor. Regardless of how extreme the various cases may be, there is always someone who is still able to play and to laugh. And humor itself has a strong therapeutic value. According to my personal definition, humor, in its truest sense, is based on tender feelings. Humor presupposes love and understanding for its target. Humor never hurts because it has compassion for its object. It certainly seems that when I demonstrate a patient's physical manifestation *humorously*, he is confronted by an affectionate and amusing image of himself. The stinging seriousness of his conflict appears to be lessened, and for the time being at least, he doesn't have to defend himself against something when that "something" strikes him as funny. In the grey setting of a mental ward, where reactions are so often alien to us, it is acutely refreshing to hear a normally anticipated response—the explosion of spontaneous laughter. In many ways, humor brings a new perspective to a patient's problem by lighting it from another side.

**I demonstrate humorously**

If humor can reach wholesome areas—still intact in most of the patients—dance has an infinitely greater therapeutic capacity. At all times, dance addresses itself directly to the healthy

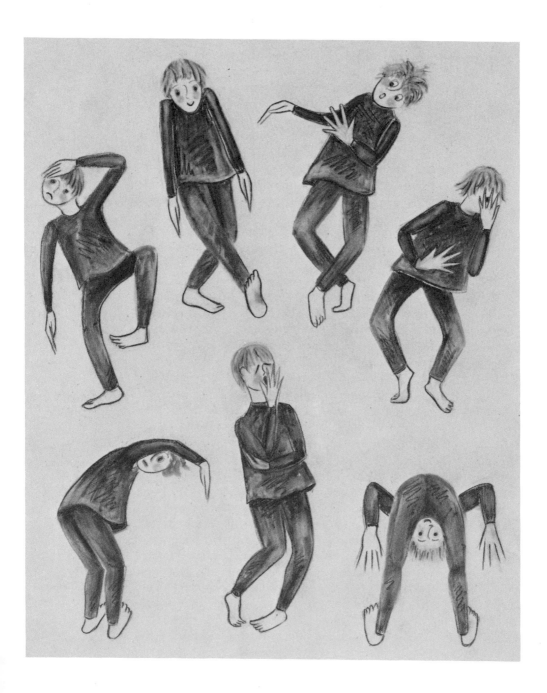

aspect of human nature and it can fortify and expand any remaining sparks of well-being. Dance assumes the natural capability of the body to move. Human movement is synonymous with life, and dance includes all of the innate elements of movement. However limited these elements have become, *somewhere* in a person their potential exists. We can and do draw upon this dormant source.

I'm sure that anyone who has experienced the world of dance knows how much pleasure the body can and should give us; knows that it demands an enjoyable participation in existence; and knows that a body in a state of well-being can counteract and counterbalance the impacts of life. Most of us can recall times when we have revelled in the sheer delight of our physical selves. But if anything happened to blight such pleasure, the victim is likely to forget the pleasure and only remember the blight. As I observe the patients I work with, it's easy to see that there's no delight in their bodies. So my immediate concern is to revive the body's talent to enjoy itself, to attempt to heal the emotional wound by inducing in the person a new and positive feeling about his physical self.

To reaffirm the innate, functional properties of the body, and to foster the healthy development of growth, I try to cover the whole range of human action from infancy to adulthood. We follow the baby's first groping explorations with the enjoyable re-experiencing of all normal childhood movements: crawling, creeping, rolling, rocking, walking, running, hopping, jumping, skipping, turning, and so on. In this primary stage, I don't set standards. I'm interested only in the patient's exploration of his own self, in his earliest physical identity. He must renew his initial development with no interference. He must be free to make his own investigations, however stumblingly. As the patient engages in elementary actions common to us all, he necessarily discovers the person who performs them: himself. He gets the first glimmer of the being he is. He begins to comprehend that **Childhood movements** this body which is crawling, hopping, and running belongs to him: *he is this body.* Very pleasurably, the patient's range of movement has been widened, and with it there emerges a first faint image of himself.

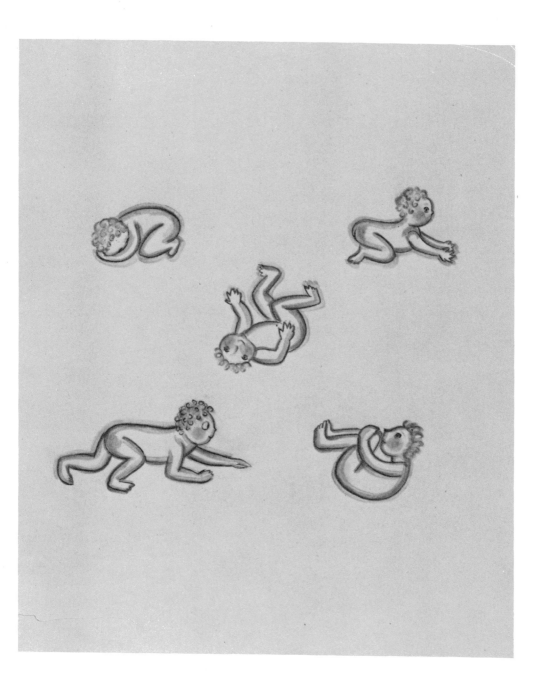

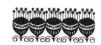

*Part 2*

# *ELEMENTS OF MOVEMENT*

Note: Human expression, as it is represented by the body, is my source of psychological evaluation. Alignment, centrality, tension, rhythm, use of space: these basic elements of movement and all their related aspects combine to create body-expression. Though these components operate simultaneously and are inextricably interwoven, I do try to separate them for the purpose of body-analysis.

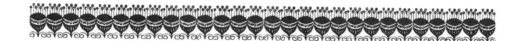

# BREATHING
## Do Only Animals Pant?

I cannot begin my discussion of dance elements without mentioning the one aspect of existence that applies to everything we do: man breathes! His first breath escorts him into life. His last breath accompanies his departure from it. And in the interim, the way he lives affects his breathing, and the way he breathes affects his living. Disordered breathing goes hand in hand with illness, mental or physical.

Functional breathing enhances the expression of the body by conforming to its feeling: the sharp intake of air in surprise or fear, the heavy expulsion of air in sobs of grief, the deep, rhythmic breathing of love, the full, fluid breathing of joy. Similarly, our breathing can adjust in various ways to expedite our every action; it adjusts rhythmically to the tempo of our running or walking. It releases with our bodies in a push or a bend. It sustains an intake of air to lighten our bodies for a jump or a leap. Breathing actively and effectively assists whatever action or feeling the body undertakes.

The patients' respiratory disturbances are displayed in many, many forms. I see staccato inhalations that sound like little, airy sobs, followed by almost imperceptible exhalations. I see individuals who close their throats in the middle of a great gulp of air, so that they choke and begin to panic. There are people whose deflated lungs carry only enough air to sustain life, and others whose chests are pumped up with great quantities of unreleased air. For the latter, exhaling is a terrifying procedure that seems to threaten loss of control or abandonment of self.

Breathing problems are not only a manifestation of acute mental disturbance. To a lesser degree but with as many variations, my regular students have similar difficulties in synchronizing their breathing with their physical or emotional states. I always wonder why there seems to be an undercurrent of embarrassment whenever the body is "out of breath." We try to hide our heaving chests, try to silence sounds escaping from them, try to maintain a facade of composure until our faces turn crimson and veins bulge out on our temples. Are we endeavoring to prove that we're in such fantastic physical shape that we never get out of breath? Or is the exhibition of normally accelerated respiration still another of our social taboos? Do only animals pant?

Wherever I look, there's so much unfunctional breathing going on, that in every class, whatever the theme and whoever the pupils, I always stress breathing and its effective application. In any way I can, I try to show pupils how to use breathing to help rather than hinder their activities, to aid, not inhibit, their emotional expression. Animal nature replaces civilized behavior when I encourage my students to run, jump, leap, until the air rushes in and out of their lungs in exhilarating gusts. I emphasize the positive aspect of this experience as well as the feeling of vigorous enjoyment that it evokes. Because it *is* a joy to sense that life-giving substance ebbing and flowing within one's body. What a miraculous function is this breathing, as it works unfailingly to support our existence!

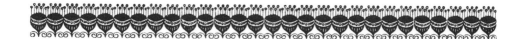

# ALIGNMENT
# A Body with a Point of View

I feel that it is most significant how our bodies are carried—how we stand on this earth. I believe that a person's body-design should ideally represent his affirmation of being, reflect the highest form of functional existence, realize a neutral, alert attitude from which he can easily act and react. It should indicate a free, adaptable body that is capable of choice and decision, a body with a point of view.

Is a person's carriage straight or crooked? Is his body rooted or aloof? Can he stand on his own two feet, or is he a leaner? Does he feel himself as a harmonious unity, or does he experience himself in bits and pieces? Which bits does he hide? Which ones does he show? These are some of the questions that come to my mind when I'm considering a body's alignment.

In physical terms, my ideal body would be erect, a plumb line from the top of the head through the soles of the feet. Its various parts would fall into peaceful agreement with the whole structure, the pliant spine lending support and balance to any position and movement. The weight would be distributed according to the center of gravity, with no strain, contraction, or pressure in any area. The inner organs, circulation, respiration, and vocal expression would function freely and efficiently. Such a posture represents the most effortless carriage, and effortlessly this body can move in any direction.

Within the sessions devoted to alignment, I use any of the typical exercises designed for that purpose, working on the floor, against the walls, at the barres, and in front of the mirrors. But beyond these, there are other movement ideas that help the patient to understand more clearly what alignment really means.

Imitation is a determinative part of learning and growth, and I use it in every conceivable way. I may demonstrate various positions and movements for the patients to "try on," presenting them with contrasting images by which they can orient themselves. I copy their bodies; they copy mine, as well as others'. Doctors in the hospital, relatives at home, people on the streets —no one escapes our alignment inspection. And as the patient learns to *look* more closely, he not only discovers the actual existence of other bodies, he also realizes that their shapes are somehow unlike his own. He compares; he differentiates.

The opposite aspects of alignment can help to clarify the body's position. We do the worst walks we can think of; we use every kind of ridiculous, overdone posture and gait, parading across the room pigeon-toed, splay-footed, knock-kneed, bow-legged. We waddle and clomp and mince. We enthusiastically make different parts of our anatomies stick out, sag, or flap. Then, when we try to walk our best, we find that it's not so easy. Some of those same distortions that we thought were so funny are disrupting our own postures. We can feel them there; they make us feel awkward, and we'd like to get rid of them!

When the patients work with partners on alignment, alternating the roles of "teacher" and "pupil," I discover much more about each one. What about "teacher's" own body? Can it demonstrate what he is trying to teach? Often he is much too easily pleased with his "pupil's" stance. Doesn't he see what's wrong with it? Maybe he hopes to get from the world the same sort of

approval he is giving. Or perhaps he's justifying his own deviations so that he can stay just as he is. And the "pupil"—how does
he respond to criticism? Is he over-anxious to agree, or does the
correction infuriate him? Is he a "compulsive student," or is he
driven to usurp the role of the teacher? Does either one of them
gain any posture-insight at all? This simple procedure of setting
the body to rights can give rise to a wide variety of reactions.
Some people quit; some think it's silly; some get embarrassed.
And even such small corrections as raising a head, straightening
an arm, or lowering a heel may be met with strong resentment
on the part of the patient, as he violently defends his unfunctional position.

# *Johnny*

Johnny's reaction was the most impressive I've ever witnessed
within the context of alignment. A deeply disoriented patient, he
had been working in my group for several months with no de-
tectable change. All the sessions on alignment and all my efforts
to induce the image of a functional walk seemed to have been
in vain. He still moved along with a "pregnant walk," his whole
body slanted so strongly backward that he constantly looked as
though he were going to fall. Only his head, thrust far forward,
attempted to compensate for the imbalance. Stiff and energetic,
his legs lifted themselves from the thigh, with feet rigidly fixed.
His arms seemed to have no volition of their own. Hanging loose
and lifeless, they were flung helplessly into the air with the force
of his militant stride.

One day, I decided to film the patients' walks. As the
orderlies were setting up the camera, I explained its unaccustomed presence:

"Today, we're going to make a movie. You can all be in it
if you want. Later next week we'll watch it together. All you'll
have to do is walk from here . . . to here . . . and back again, one
at a time. Please try to feel easy; just walk naturally."

It was astonishing to see some of the most unresponsive and
withdrawn patients suddenly beginning to behave like prima

donnas fighting for a star spot! In spite of my request for natural behavior, they all tried to impress the camera. Curiously enough, their apparent efforts to "walk well" resulted in the further exaggeration of each individual's habitual alignment disturbance. I watched, fascinated, as the film recorded a chin poked far out, a painfully contracted spinal arch, a flailing arm, a hiked-up chest, a flapping foot. And as for Johnny, every nuance of his unusual gait was prominently projected.

A week later we ran the film, presenting the men with their own moving pictures. Johnny's reaction to the incontestible evidence of his walk was immediate and explosive. He grabbed my hand and shouted:

"No! That's not me! I *don't* walk like that! Oh, Jesus, that's *awful!*"

And when the film was over he wouldn't leave the room. He wanted to see himself again—hoping, perhaps, that his eyes had deceived him the first time. When he came to the session the next morning, Johnny still looked shaken, but it soon became clear that he was determined to fight for a change. And sure enough, the wonder occurred. In fourteen days a new body emerged. Properly aligned, standing straight and firm on the earth, Johnny's attitude toward himself and toward life had joined his body in a remarkable transformation.

I believe that Johnny's striking response was due to the confrontation with his entire self in action, probably for the first time in his life. Though he had seemingly ignored the many sessions on posture correction, *some* aspects of harmonious alignment must have registered; otherwise he wouldn't have been able to see the difference, and wouldn't have felt the urge to change.

To me, the fact that Johnny was filmed in a walk is significant. A walk is the most universal mode of travel, the simplest way for the human to transport himself from one place to another. Barring physical handicaps, we all can walk. The question is "HOW?" The manner of a person's walk is as individual as his thumbprint. In no other action is his alignment so clearly revealed. In no other way does he display himself so emphatically.

**Johnny**

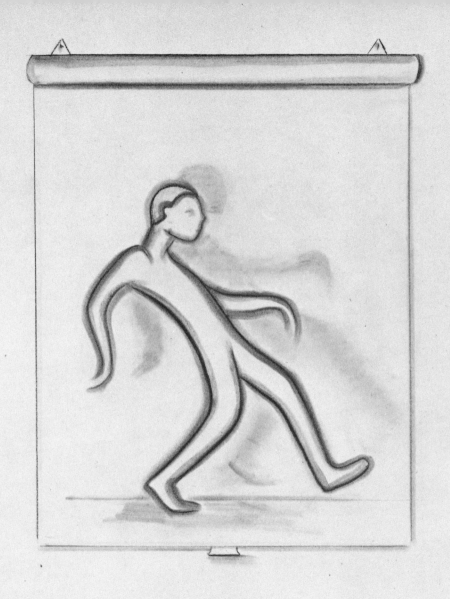

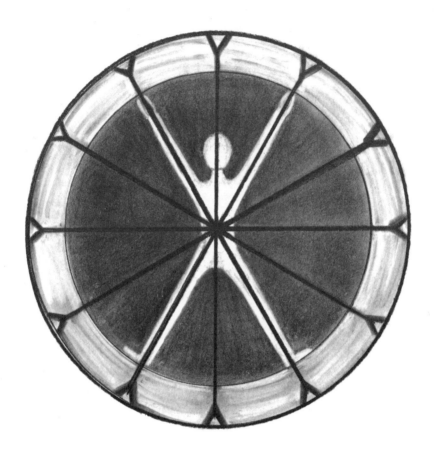

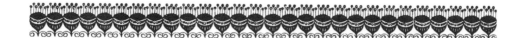

# CENTER

## *His Middle Bespeaks the Man*

The center is precisely what the word indicates: the middle area of the human form. It is the center that makes physical and emotional unity possible. Acting as the stabilizer for our equilibrium, the compass for our orientation, the coordinator for our movement, the point of reference that defines our physical boundaries, it tells us where we begin and where we end. My work has been considerably supported by my belief that the center is the physical equivalent of the human self. As such, it bespeaks the individual's relationship toward his own being and toward the world around him.

The muscles included in this area must be able to contract and expand for adequate response to any stimulus. When they contract, the body closes inward; when they expand, the body opens outward. Any time the body opens out or closes in, any time the person reaches and retrieves, pushes or pulls, the action emanates from the center. Actually, the body has no other alternative; every movement goes either toward or away from the

**Center**

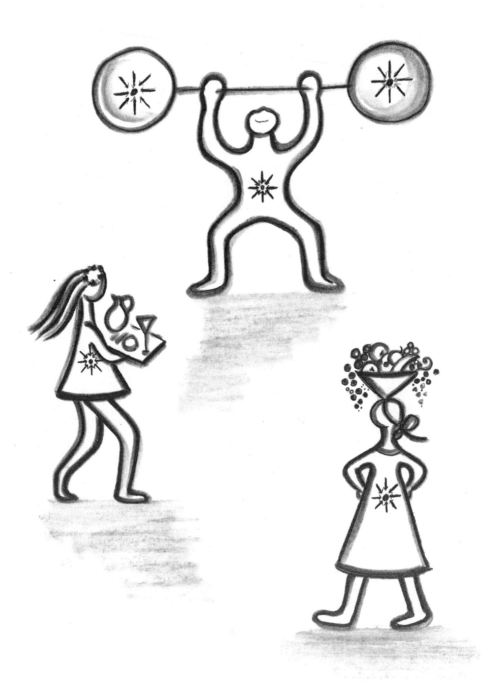

center, just as every feeling is directed toward or away from the self.

How aptly we describe our feelings in terms of the body, and particularly in terms of the center! "Gut-level reactions," "sinking feelings in the pit of the stomach," "belly laughs," "intestinal fortitude," "My stomach's all tied up in knots!"—in our common speech, the center bespeaks the emotional man.

However the center responds to whatever feeling, it instantly prepares the body for action. When we witness a crass injustice, righteous indignation causes our "stomachs to churn" as all our energies join forces in this vital spot; our legs are made ready to run for the police, or our backs to turn from the scene, or our bodies and arms to lash out in attack against the offender. As soon as our action is concluded and the feeling expended, the center returns to its neutral state, where it awaits the next call to action. The center seems to be the starting and the ending point for the body's behavior. As such, it allows for functional balance between feeling and action, between inner and outer existence.

At different times, we find that we can temporarily stress either the "in" or the "out." If we want to concentrate, meditate, refuel our energies, we can shut out any environmental distraction, whether it's a beautiful sunset or the racket of a riveting machine. Just as effectively, we can become completely involved in what is going on around us, surrendering ourselves to the beauty of nature or concerning ourselves with the needs of others. Back and forth we swing, giving as well as taking, listening as well as talking, controlling or letting go, accepting or refusing, experiencing the world and allowing the world to experience us.

Occasionally we can see this fluctuation disrupted, as when a person continually emphasizes either of the two possibilities. The primarily inner-directed person may be characterized as introverted, unworldly, anti-social, or, most aptly, self-centered.

**Stabilizer for our equilibrium**

Whatever he's called, his body is inclined to close in and shut out. We see shuttered eyes, folded arms, squeezed-together thighs. He's a poor listener, hard to reach. Preoccupied with his own person, he's interested in outside events only as they relate to himself. Anything that anyone says is perceived as though it

93

were meant to affect him alone. He is the center of the world, around which everyone else and everything else must revolve. He is unable or unwilling to relate to anyone else's world.

The person who is "sold on the world" is usually labelled extroverted, flighty, or superficial. His whole body is outward bound; its every action is exteriorized. But he's just as difficult to reach as our introverted friend. Though he's talkative and convivial, he remains quite noncommittal about his own being. He may give bits of himself to many, but he can't commit himself fully to any one person or any one thing. In both cases, we see isolated, lonely human beings: one a fugitive from the world, the other a refugee from the self.

Lopsided as our introvert and extrovert may be, at least they know which direction they want to take. They've settled on a particular identity, and they like it that way. But there are so many others who don't seem to know who they are (at least that's what they tell me). From encounter groups to marathons to such splinter activities as partner swapping and candle-lit dinners-in-the-nude, a large part of the citizenry is engaged in an all-out hunt for the "real me." Has "reason for being" been smothered in the crush of overpopulation? Have the endless war years driven the self into the comparative safety of anonymity? Or is it just easier for someone to say, "I don't know who I am" and avoid all responsibility for his actions? Whatever has brought a person to this distressing condition, his nebulous self can still be glimpsed in his body's wishy-washy center. Its devitalized muscles advertise the weakness of their housing. Without impetus from that center, its owner's movements are vague. His speech is inarticulate whenever he voices his indecisive thoughts. And his feelings . . . where are they?

Under any severe emotional stress, even the most well-adjusted person can be thrown off-balance temporarily, and lose his sense of self. In the throes of panic or anguish, the center is thrown into chaos, discharging energy every which way. Movements become disorganized, breathing turns to gasping, speech is incoherent; the whole body is disoriented, in turmoil. As the person escapes from an unbearable reality, he is the picture of self-disintegration. But in this case, when the reaction is lived through, the center regains its control, and operates to restore emotional and physical equilibrium.

When I visited the ward that first day, the patients had seemed like "empty shells." No one appeared to be home in any of the human forms I talked with. The person's self seemed to be in absentia. What, exactly, were those bodies doing to give me such an uncanny impression?

I discovered that I was reacting to fragmented pieces of bodies rather than their whole forms. A fist, a foot, an eyebrow was making such an overwhelming statement of its own that it overshadowed the person it belonged to. The isolated part was serving as a substitute center. . . .

I saw unanchored bodies: weightless, suspended, avoiding gravity, slanting perilously into space. . . .

And there was the man in constant movement, running without direction in everlasting flight. . . .

There were those who had drawn back into themselves lying fetus-like on the floor, locked in their own stillness. . . .

I remember the one whose eyes had stared into limitless space; and the other, gazing deep into his inmost recesses. Unforgettable, those eyes . . .

These were the patients whose bodies represented the epitome of fragmentation, the absolute of one-sided orientation, the ultimate in loss of center and self.

# Frances

I took the girl's hand, stepped back so that our arms were extended, and asked her to pull me toward her. She just stared at me.

"What do you mean? Toward where?"

"Toward you," I repeated.

"But where shall I . . . HOW? How can I?"

"Just bend your elbow, Frances, and pull on my hand. Pull me toward yourself."

Long did she look at me, then tried desperately to do as I asked, pulling me first to one side, then to the other, then high

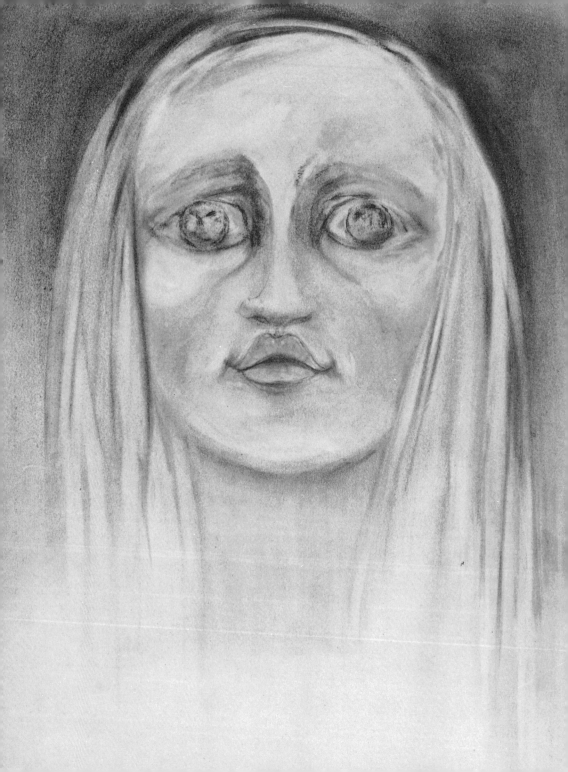

up, then way down to the floor. But she just couldn't find the "you" I wanted to be pulled toward. Since she didn't know where her self was, she had no way of relating *me* to *it*.

# Carrie and Diane

As I begin to work for the restoration of a functional center, I usually apply every anatomical exercise I can think of that will bring its particular muscles into play. I ask for contractions and releases in the whole circumference of the centric area. I want the patients to feel how these muscles can initiate the opening and closing of their bodies. It's easier said than done. . . .

There was Carrie. A heavy-set girl with a flabby belly, she commenced to cry:

"I can't find any muscles in my stomach! Where are they? What are you talking about?"

I applied gentle pressure on her abdomen so she could feel where the action would be, but she slapped my hand away, sobbing:

"I don't have any, I tell you! They aren't there. Leave me alone!"

Which I did, for the time being at least. But I couldn't help thinking that her sobs were activating those muscles whether she knew it or not.

In vivid contrast to Carrie, who couldn't find her center, was Diane, who couldn't let go of it. Hard and resistant as a flatiron, her center constantly retracted upon itself. Whenever I saw her, in sessions or just standing around the ward, her arms were clamped around her middle as if she had an epic stomach-ache. In the classes, she couldn't seem to respond to any exercise that might have loosened up those center muscles. She continued to stay locked in her own embrace. One day, I took her arms and carefully tried to open them.

**Unforgettable, those eyes**

"Don't . . . don't!" she whispered in terror. "I can't let go. Don't you see? . . . I'd fall apart."

For me, the two girls represented the extremes of center

imbalance: the one unaware of her center's existence, the other preoccupied with its preservation.

When patients are so "out of their bodies" that they can't find out how or where a muscle contracts or releases, all the best exercises in the world won't do the trick. Other ways must be devised to make them conscious of their dormant centers. There are commonplace actions which can't possibly be carried through without the center's cooperation. Tug-of-war is a contest that automatically creates center-contraction as two people pull on the rope against each other's weight. Pictures can be hung on the walls as high as the patient can reach, thus insuring a good stretch for the center muscles. I may ask the group to rearrange the furniture in any way that suits them. More often than not, they willingly take on the role of interior decorator. They lift and push and pull the chairs and tables about. Carpets are rolled up and dragged from place to place. The piano is shoved across the hall, to the accompaniment of grunts, groans, much clowning around—and a lot of center contraction.

In my search for the patients' center-selves, I may work with objects or images, partners or groups. I can combine feelings and actions with the other elements of movement. Contractions can be strong or soft, fast or slow. We can close in lovingly, shyly, angrily, expand in joy, in pride, or with a good, deep breath. I can ask the class to "change a tire," "inhale a cigarette," "steal a cookie," within the structure of a rhythmical form, thereby converting these procedures into abdominal adagios. Unconventional as they may seem to be, within such "dance" sessions, dedicated to the fine art of contraction and release, the performers suddenly begin to get the message. Martha Graham would be proud of us!

Just as one can't conceive of boundaries without some sort of center, it's also impossible to imagine a center without some sort of boundaries. But implicit in every patient's center disturbance is the apparent nonexistence of his physical outline. He looks and acts as if he doesn't know where he begins or where he ends. He seems to have no clear image of his body as a whole, nor can he recognize his body parts as being portions of himself.

**Martha Graham
would be proud of us**

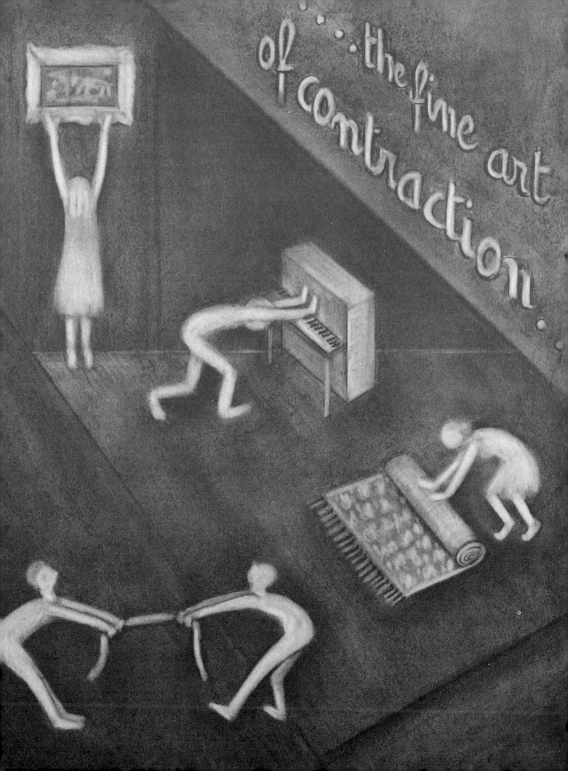

...the fine art of contraction...

Though he has been conditioned by the hospital routine to perform certain necessary functions, he doesn't appear to realize that the body which walks, feeds, sits, and lies down for him, *actually is himself.*

The body informs the human about the world around him, but the self must be present to receive that information. Only a person's sense of identity can determine whether his body is coming or going, starting or stopping. And only when an individual can distinguish his own being as different from the being of a tree, a cat, a stove, or a mother, can he recognize himself.

I use every available means to give the body back to its owner. We begin by investigating our own bodies, every part of them, just as we once explored them in infancy. Often a patient looks at his hand or his foot as if he were seeing it for the first time. As he feels his own body with his own hands, and strokes along its outlines, he begins to perceive it as a substance with a shape and texture and temperature.

# Linda

Linda didn't seem to know where her head was; at least it was the most obviously neglected part of her, with its tangled hair and grimy face. As we worked together, I noticed that she couldn't ever manage to find her face, although she could locate every other part of her anatomy. Her hands would approach its general direction but would always stop in the air, a good twelve inches from each cheek. It looked as if she were feeling a huge head perched up there on top of her thin little neck. I wanted her to discover its realistic size for herself, but I had to make up a game to trick her into it. We sat on the floor, aiming to touch face, hips, knees, feet—in the same progression, over and over again. And feet, knees, and hips were firmly grasped, but whenever it came time for the face, Linda's hands halted, as usual, in the air. So I gradually increased the tempo of the pattern until the action was going so fast that she lost control of her "brake." Suddenly, her hands clapped solidly on each cheek. She remained frozen in this position, her horrified eyes staring at me.

Then she began to cry, loudly and steadily, until the class was over. But her stormy reaction was followed by quite a change. She was absent from the next few sessions. But one day there she stood in the doorway, her hair washed and brushed, her face scrubbed clean, and her lips painted a bright red. And from that time on, Linda touched her face whenever I asked, with no signs of distress whatsoever.

When the body's outline and all of its parts are accounted for, it is time to relate them to the center, to identify them as extensions of the self. When Eric's foot is wiggling, it is Eric who is wiggling his foot. When Rosalia's finger is poking, it is Rosalia

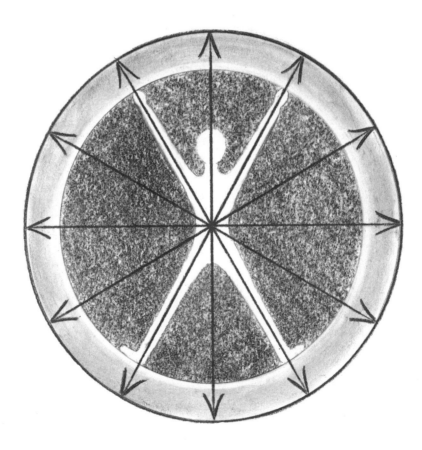

**Center**

who pokes her finger. Bill is shrugging *his* shoulders. Jean is waving *her* arm. A familiar waltz melody can bring our parts together. We hum its tune as our hands begin to swing from side to side. Then the swing includes the arms, the shoulders, the head, the upper torso, the hips, the legs . . . until the whole body is one swinging unit that declares:

"This body that swings is *mine.* . . . *I* am swinging."

Finally, each person can begin to relate his body to other human bodies. I want to clarify for Ernest where Franz begins and ends, and for Franz where Ernest begins and ends. To stress individual differences, I ask the patient to see and touch another person's body just as he learned to see and touch his own. As two partners face each other, I can give each one a different way of moving: round movements vs. angular, soft vs. staccato, slow vs. fast. Or they may show each other different expressions: silliness confronting sadness, boredom looking at happiness, anger watching friendliness. There is no end to the distinctions that can be made between the *You* and the *Me* as the patient struggles to develop a sense of identity.

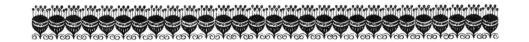

# TENSION

## *It Has to Do with Letting Go!*

In dance terminology, the word "tension" stands for a person's talent to energize and de-energize his physical being. The definition assumes that any part of the body, or the body as a whole, can play with flexible abandon within the entire range between the two possibilities.

Every one of us has his own characteristic degree of tension, the one which is the most comfortable and familiar. And it is from this basic level that we increase or decrease our energy output. Ideally, it represents a condition in which the same amount of tension is equally distributed over the entire body. Whatever the quality of the individual's natural tonicity—soft, strong, light, heavy, fluid, firm—it is unabashedly declared throughout his body. Of course, we constantly leave this state. Whatever we do, whatever we see, hear, taste, touch, smell, whatever we think or dream, our reactions to life cause our tension to increase or decrease. But when the reaction is completed, our tension again becomes harmoniously attuned.

As we watch a person react, it becomes most apparent that increasing tension parallels feeling-intensification, just as decreasing tension parallels feeling-abatement. Ideally, the two rise together, reach consummation together, and descend together. This process permits an action to be fulfilled and an emotion to achieve its natural climax. If a person blocks either the feeling or the action in its ascendency, he will never know the gratification of fulfillment. He will forever seek an experience he has denied himself.

Tension disturbances are many and varied. Let's look at a few of the more obvious ones, beginning with the individual who is addicted to only one gradation of the tension scale. Most easily visualized is the person who is dedicated to either of its extremes:

Mr. Tense: Body always "on the go"
        Movements abrupt, hasty
        Muscles contracted
        Attitude of overwhelming intensity
        In constant competition with himself and his
            world
        Motto: "It's later than you think!"

Mr. Loose: Spongy physique
        Slothful in body
        Passive in soul
        Attitude of boredom
        Confuses relaxing with collapsing
        Motto: "Mañana."

Although any of us may have the tendency to overemphasize one extreme or the other, we are certainly capable of adaptation whenever necessary. To continue to live, we must sleep, however fitfully. We must move about, however languidly. But in the wards of mental hospitals are individuals for whom there is no longer any possibility for adaptation. One aspect of tension is represented in their bodies as a permanent fixation. These patients eat, work, and speak within the prison of their tension. Their armor is imprinted with its causative emotion. We see not an angry man, but a frozen *symbol* of rage; not a sorrowing woman, but an *emblem* of despair.

**It hurts right here**

It is interesting that tension so often has the connotation of *tenseness*, which to the dancer represents only one degree of tension. But this particular degree is the one which concerns me most, since it demonstrates muscular conflict created by a mental conflict.

Whenever energy accumulates in one part of the body, it sets up a roadblock in the path of the normal flow of energy. Most people are well aware of these "stop signs" in their bodies and are fascinated by them. Ask anyone where his tension spot lies, and he'll gladly present a fifteen-minute dissertation on the subject. He will describe in minute detail its exact location, its precise degree, and the inconvenience it causes him. It may be a tense right shoulder, a stiff neck, a knotted stomach, a cramp in the left little toe, or a problem with teeth-grinding. But the minute I begin to make helpful suggestions which entail altering his self-image, up come the defenses!

"But I've always tilted my head to one side. That's just me!"

"But I don't want to relax my pelvis. I'd look like a tramp!"

"But what's wrong with my spine? Everybody raves about my posture!"

Whether they want to change their appearance or not, most people are eager to have their specialty-in-tension interpreted:

"Really now, why *do* I pull my shoulders up? I mean—what do they say to you? Why do *you* think I do it?"

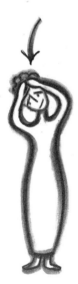
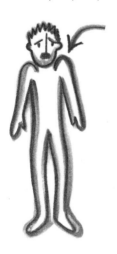
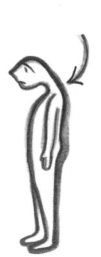
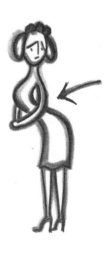

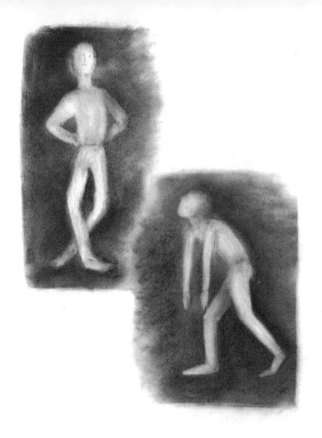

**Split figures**

My only reply can be, "I honestly don't know—you could pull them up for many reasons. But I do see your shoulders saying to me, 'Please help us to relax!' And for now, that's just what we should try to do."

How long the way can be from the first recognition of a tension "hangup" to its full correction! The person seems to cling to his unfunctional body statement even when he's fully aware of the unnecessary amount of energy it requires, even, sometimes, after he's recalled its psychological origin, and even though it hurts. But I've found out that *if* the symptomatic tension can be released, its causative mental conflict stands a good chance of being resolved. That's what is so great about dance therapy: when we deal with the physical symptom, we're dealing directly with the feeling that created it.

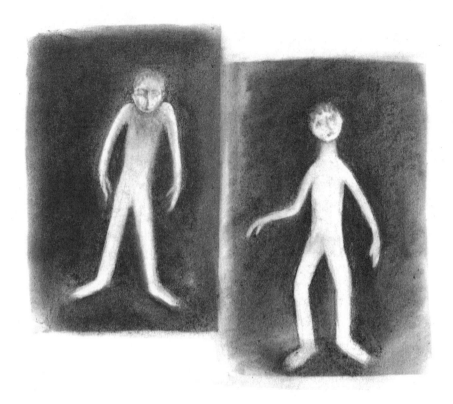

It was while I was watching some of my patients that I first became aware of their magnified versions of our little stop signs. And I remembered Bleuler talking about "Die Spaltung"—"The Split." I was now seeing in the schizophrenic body the term he used to define the schizophrenic mind. They were split in tension; they were split in expression. Soft, smiling face was mounted on stiff, stubborn body. Angry, contracted feet belied tender, limp hands. A boldly thrust out chest loomed over a weak, collapsed pelvis. These separations seem to occur in every element of movement, or in any combination of elements. Wherever they exist, they forcefully characterize the set, divided expression of the patient's divided mind.

Whether over- or under-energized, those massive fixations must be broken up. The first assault is made very gently, with childhood movements. Even the earliest ones, like crawling or rolling, bring unused areas of the body into play so that tension changes are bound to occur. Animation of one body part at a time isolates each of them, so that the patient can become aware of them. We articulate each joint, activate heads, hands, arms— any portion of ourselves that can be consciously activated. Faces grimace, hands shake, fingers wiggle, feet tap, toes wriggle; hips can flounce, heads can toss, bodies can tumble. These actions can be combined with other movements in a limitless variety of ways. Gradually, chinks begin to appear in the patient's armor. The blocked form starts to come apart as its segments are freed from its whole.

Every human must constantly cope with situations that demand different degrees of tension. If a mother, carrying her infant over an icy pavement, would employ the same amount of energy in her arms that she must use in her center and legs, she'd crush her baby's ribs! We split ourselves up in similar ways countless times a day, without even being aware of it.

For this reason, I purposely create split tensions in the bodies of my patients to make them conscious of what they are doing unconsciously. Energy-splitting can become quite a hilarious game, more difficult than you might think when it has to be done intentionally. In the course of a session, I may pick up split-body conditions that are being manifested by members of the group, or I may rely on my own collection of "standard splits." We can move around with tight, contracted faces and sloppy, slack bodies, or skip with "rag-doll" arms and stiff "wooden" legs, or run with one whole side rigid and the other side loose. Some people seem to understand better if I call the splits by feeling-names. We greet each other with a happy face and a sad body, or a brave chest with a scared pelvis; or we say goodbye with an obstinate right side and a sentimental left side. We try to say "yes" with our heads, "no" with our hands, and "maybe" with our feet. Certainly it sounds ridiculous. But it's the very absurdity of the exaggerations that make them fun for the patients to do.

The eventual mastery of body-splitting seems to create for anyone a sense of self-control and satisfaction; just as we, as children, felt so proud when we could finally rub our stomachs at the same time we patted our heads; and just as the pianist gains a feeling of triumph when he can play pianissimo with his right hand, while his left hand performs a ponderous forté.

The very word "separation" presupposes the potential of unity, just as the word "unity" presupposes the potential of separation. Thus, my sessions on tension-splitting have served as a prelude to the realization of unified tension.

So, once I have pulled the body to pieces, I have to put it back together again, not as a calcified block, but as a fluid unanimity with every body part in mutual agreement. As a beginning, I've found it best to work from the two extremes of tension. Almost anyone can grasp the idea of tightness or looseness, and can make himself stiff, or limp all over, and then jump, or run, or dance about. When the patients are well acquainted with those two extreme possibilities, then they can be introduced to the degrees that lie between them. From the tightest, I can then ask for less . . . less . . . still less . . . and finally, least. And from the loosest, more . . . more . . . still more . . . and finally, most. The body becomes more flexible as the patient practices the tension scale, and the patient can find the one degree in which his body feels most comfortable. He discovers his functional, basic level of energy.

At last the whole body is ready to experience one degree of tension, sustain one level of energy throughout. To capture this oneness, I can adapt the entire body's tension to the tension in one of its parts. Starting with a clenched fist, for example, we lead the tension being felt by the hand into the whole arm. We move it across the chest and shoulders—involving the head en route—and down into the other arm. It is then spread downward through torso, legs, and feet, until the entire body feels like a fist. This progression can be initiated by any portion of the body, in any degree of tension. In the same way, the whole body's energy level can be matched to a joyful face, a nervous foot, an aggressive chest, a boisterous shout. It's really astonishing how these maneuvers are able to create in a body the harmonious unity that is so vital for competent performance.

The collaboration of emotional urgency and maximum energy can produce phenomenal results. There was the woman who lifted a car up and away from the body of her child who lay pinned beneath it. Motivated by a single need, her energy directed to a single action, she became endowed with such superhuman strength that she was able to perform a miraculous feat. Of course, that's a classic example. But it does seem that success in any undertaking, whether it be plowing a field or conducting a symphony, can be most effectively achieved with the unified cooperation of energy and feeling, involved in the pursuit of a single goal.

How fervently I wish to instill the capacity for such total involvement. So many of us consistently control the deed, edit the thought, stifle the emotion, long before it can reach consummation. Since tension increases with the intensification of involvement, I know that I can intensify involvement by increasing tension. I must try to bring about unbroken, mounting energy in the body until it reaches fulfillment, then allow it to diminish, unbroken, to its natural basic level. This pattern of rising . . . climaxing . . . falling will grant my wish for fulfillment.

We use any of the elements of dance, singly or in combination, as we work with the rise and fall of energy to further a patient's involvement. We can make any gesture bigger and bigger. We can move in little space, in more space, in a lot of space. We can move faster and faster, progressing from a stroll to a walk to a trot to a race. Or we can increase tension and involvement by intensifying our interest in any object. It captures our attention; we become more intrigued . . . fascinated . . . absorbed . . . spellbound. We may find the object unusual . . . amusing . . . funny . . . hilarious.

However we go about it, the climax is sustained for the amount of time that's needed to experience it fully. Understandably, the duration of this peak experience varies considerably from person to person.

But, of course, whatever goes up must come down. After the peak, we reverse the pattern. However we increased tension and involvement, we return by the same path to our original point of departure. Affect and energy diminish together as we become slower and slower, smaller and smaller, less and less interested. Certainly, lowering our level of energy is just as important to a balanced existence as raising it; and if consummation has been realized, we can descend easily to our normal level of functioning.

But it's quite another matter if the climax was only partially attained. We're left hanging in the air, and residues of affect and energy go astray. Some people relieve themselves in frustrated dog-kicking or child-swatting; but most of us, I believe, instinctively allow our bodies to release that remaining excitation in less hurtful and more productive ways. A walk around the block, beating the rugs, washing the car, ten laps up and down the pool—any strong action will expend any left-over tensions and cut them down to size.

When at last the collaboration of tension and involvement has been attained, the patient can experience himself and his actions as a coordinated unity. He can then afford to share himself with another person. Two bodies can become one unified partnership as they increase and decrease a rhythmic movement pattern together. They move, feel, grow together, and encounter the heights together. And I've noticed that after they've decreased the action and regained their separate identities, a new element has been added to their relationship. Patients who had never paid any attention to each other before are suddenly compatible; they'll sit down together at meals, play ping-pong, or watch TV together. In the same way, all members of the group can develop a new relationship as they join forces in projecting a common idea, action, or feeling, intensifying and reducing it in unison. Though each person is supporting the concept of a single goal, the realization of his own contribution can strengthen his sense of identity.

Major changes can occur in the patient if these concepts are applied over a long period of time. His energy level will be more equable, his coordination improved, his concentration span increased. He'll know something about "getting his steam up" as well as letting it simmer down—and when and how to do both.

We find our "tension specialists" in the field of athletics: the ski-jumper, the high-diver, and especially the pole-vaulter, whose body most specifically designs the pattern of rising, climaxing, and falling. His tension mounts in the running preparation,

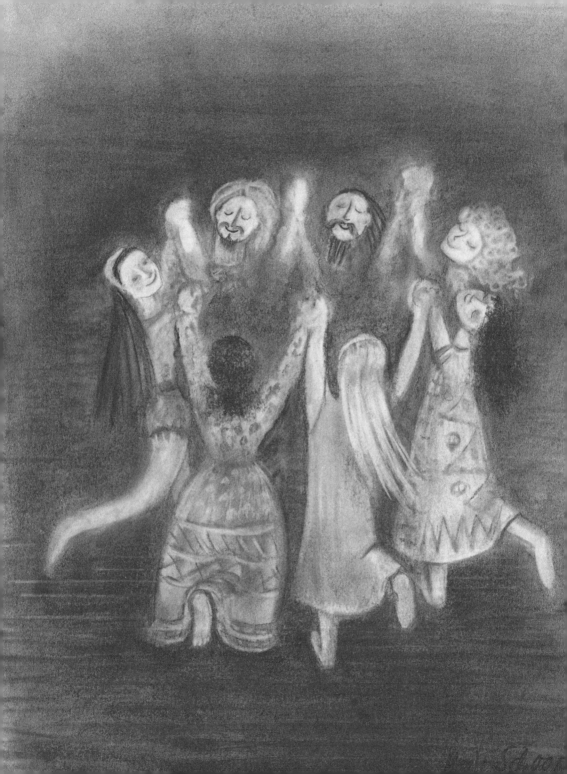

reaches its optimum in the lift and twist over the bar, then releases in every muscle for the tumble to the ground.

Have you ever seen the great folk ballets, the dancers from the Soviet Union, Mexico, Greece, Israel . . . ? Have you ever participated in a folk dance yourself? It's an experience not to be missed. Excitement builds to an exhilarating frenzy as the turns, the stamping, the clapping, the intricate patterns become faster and faster. The gestures become stronger, sharper, the human involvement more intense, until spirit, music, and dancers all reach a spectacularly joyous and unified finale. Then lawyer, teenager, housewife, sculptor—the whole heterogeneous crowd at the local cafe—release their excitement in a chorus of panting, uninhibited, happy exhaustion.

What a sense of fulfillment can be derived from experiences such as these! Lovers know this feeling, or women in childbirth.

And the same pattern of flux and reflux manifests itself as we live out our lives: we grow, reach the pinnacle of our years, and decline to their end. It's *how* we do it that counts.

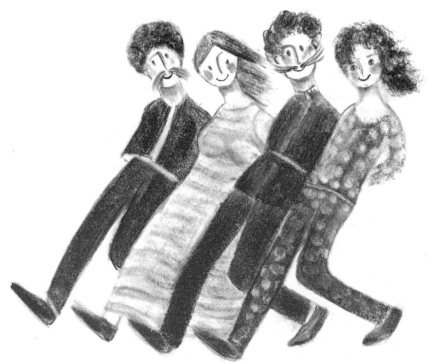

**Folk dancing**

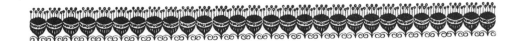

# RHYTHM
## The Battle of the Beat

In rhythmic intervals, day follows night, and night follows day; the oceans ebb and flow. Spring, summer, autumn, and winter come and go. Suns, moons, and stars orbit in eternal cadences. Birth and death compose the rhythmic patterns of man's history; breath and heartbeat are the metric elements of his life. Our language is rhythm. Rhythm is our work, our play, our song, and our dance.

Every one of us is included in the universal rhythm, and I can't believe that there is any one person in this world who is not a part of it. Yet, whenever I introduce rhythmical exercises in my classes, at least one student will desperately explain to me that he never could, and never will be able to follow a beat.

## Halacz

I'm convinced that there must be an underlying psychological reason for anyone's inability to follow a rhythm. Halacz was the first to bolster this conviction. He was a member of my first performing group. A competent dancer, attractive, with an instinctive talent for mimicry, he would have been a tremendous asset, except that he seemed to be devoid of any sense of rhythmical structure. In rehearsals and in performances he would come down from a leap too soon, begin a turn too late. He'd emphasize the wrong beat and swing his arm around a waist on the wrong note. His poor timing drove the other dancers crazy; they deluged me with complaints. On stage, they often pushed him angrily into what we called the "right rhythmical pronunciation." Off stage, he was given the cold shoulder by his fellow artists. I knew I had to do something about the situation—fast.

It occurred to me that Halacz was a rhythmical paradox. In our daily training sessions he improvised beautiful rhythmic patterns of his own. They were by no means primitive; they were long combinations of intricate tempo changes. So one day, I asked him to give the group a lesson in rhythm. My suggestion stunned the dancers at first; then they burst out laughing. As the session progressed, however, the laughter stopped. He took over with authority, and all those versatile dancers were engrossed in trying to do what Halacz did. They couldn't. That night at the performance, we all watched Halacz with renewed hope. We were soon disappointed. His leap landed too early. His turn began too late. He stood in the wings, still painstakingly counting to himself, long after his entrance cue. His timing was still all wrong.

One night after the show, Halacz and I had supper together, and he began to tell me about his childhood.

"My father was a tremendous man with immense bushy whiskers. He was a real health buff, and seemed to be dedicated to bringing me up according to his strenuous physical regimen. He made me hike with him for miles and miles. I'll never forget the length of his stride. Much as I would try to stretch my legs, I still had to take four steps to his one. But our pace was inflexible and Father set it to suit himself. I remember how I used to worry about not being able to keep up. How mad Father would be at me! Maybe he'd just leave me there alone on the mountain . . . it really scared the hell out of me.

"When at long last we'd stop for a rest, it was time for deep breathing exercises. 'Inhale for six counts,' he'd shout, 'like this!' I can still see his great hairy chest expanding to the bursting point. 'Then hold it—like this!' His face would grow purple. 'Now exhale for six counts!' And all that air rushed out again in a torrent. He sure was a tough act to follow!"

"I wonder, Halacz," I began cautiously. "You know, when you told me that story just now you *still* looked frightened. Do you think you're still fighting with him, with his domineering authority, especially the rhythmical part of it? I mean, if you're still opposing him, then maybe that's why you can't follow the rhythms of my choreography. . . ."

Halacz stared at me, scowling. After a long silence, he said, "I'll have to think about that one. . . . I don't know, maybe you're right. But I do know that I can't keep up with your beats any more than I could keep up with my father's. Actually, it's infuriating to have to adjust to either one of you!"

It certainly seemed that Halacz had discovered the reason for his difficulty. In any case, he soon began to shed his problems with timing; and gradually, he became as rhythmically accurate in our performances as he was in his own compositions.

We can't ask the patients to verbalize their childhood traumas for our convenience. In the beginning, they can't accept a "rhythmic authority" any more than Halacz could. If it's introduced too early, they may feel that a structured rhythm is an arbitrary sort of discipline, and they'll have no part of it. They must be given ample time to use their own natural rhythms before they can follow one which is given to them.

The possibilities for rhythm instruction are limitless, so I shall mention the few that have benefitted my psychotic students in special ways.

There are the beaters: several long reeds taped together at one end to form a handle. The beater seems to be a non-threatening rhythmical tool; the person using it doesn't have to take responsibility for its behavior. It can brush or tap or swat the floor, or make designs in space. It serves as a vehicle for the emotions, allowing the patient to express feelings he normally forbids himself, all within his own rhythmic pattern. The beater acts as an extension of the self.

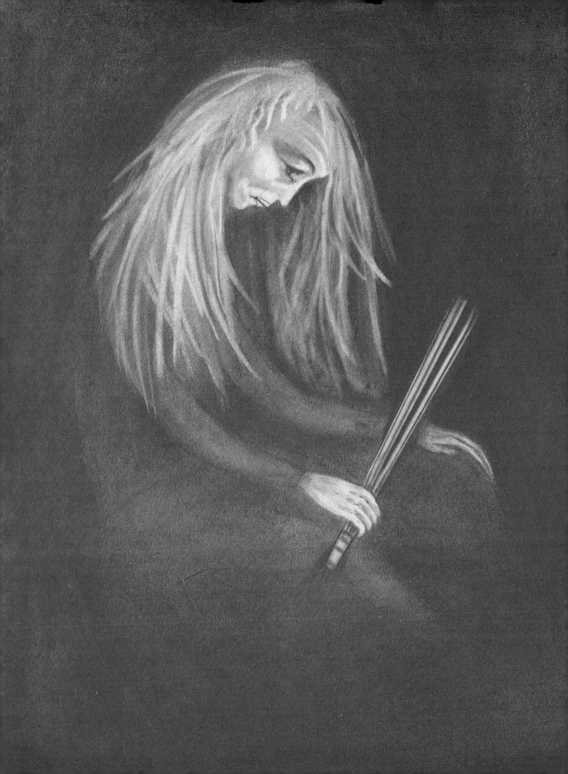

To acquaint each person with his own particular rhythmical inclination, I may ask the group to show me how they perform various daily tasks:

"How do you get up in the morning—fast or slow? Are you immediately wide-awake or do you doze off again?"

And as each one acts out his individual way of combing his hair, brushing his teeth, getting dressed, or working at his assigned tasks, he can learn a great deal about his entire rhythmic set-up. For as long as necessary, the patients walk at their own speeds, clap their own rhythms, stamp in their own qualities and time patterns, without being dominated by music, drum, or me.

When the person is secure within his own basic rhythm, I can begin to structure time by directing him to the beat of his own heart.

"I'd like all of you to take your pulses, like the nurses do. Feel it there in your wrist. When you're sure of its tempo, give each beat a sound; one sound for every beat. . . ."

After a while, all pulses are located, and the hall is filled with rhythmic sounds—some slower, some faster; some higher, some lower—a chorus of voices chanting the beats of their lives: "Dah-dah-dah-dah, bom-bom-bom-bom, tuk-tuk-tuk-tuk . . ." Soon the sounds even out, the fast ones slowing down and the slow ones speeding up, until all voices are sounding in unison. At that point, the drum or the pianist can take over, continuing the rhythm created by the patients themselves. When the beat is firmly established, I can ask them to move their body parts to it. The fact that they are interpreting their own rhythms, not mine, makes them enjoy the performance much more.

Next, we can move the whole body, altering its position with every count. It's amazing to see those bodies really begin to dance as they are spurred on to spontaneous changes by the rhythm they created. We can fit familiar movements to the beat, enjoying the experience of being synchronized with one another. Finally, with the addition of vocal sounds, every part of the human is involved in a unity of rhythmic expression.

When patients no longer defend themselves against the domination of a given beat, I can open up the rhythmical field. By accenting the first beat of four (or three or five or seven), we

**Woman
with beater**

organize time; we structure it. The constant repetition of a definite rhythm seems to provide a sense of security for the patients, in much the same way that children love to hear the familiar sounds of nursery rhymes or lullabies, over and over and over again. As the patients give in to the rhythm, reassured by its neutral, un-emotional authority, they learn to accept an enjoyable discipline.

From rhythmical acceptance, we can move to rhythmical disagreement. I ask the patients to oppose my steady drum beat with their beaters: faster or slower or louder—whatever way they feel like beating, as long as it goes against mine. The room clatters and swishes and slaps, a ruckus of rhythmic revolution. Then they alternate, part of the time beating with me, part of the time against me, learning to say "I wont," as well as "I will." Such exercises become more meaningful for the patient when he can create his own rhythmical combinations within a given struc-tured beat. Again the concept of balance has been presented, between adaptation and individual creation.

A juggler is a miracle man of timing as he keeps all those spinning balls and discs whirling through the air at different tempos. Why are his rhythmic splits such a pleasure to watch, and those of the patients so distressing? First, the juggler's own will determines when and how his body will fragment its rhyth-mic behavior. He is in command of its independent actions; he has created them himself for the express purpose of showing off exquisite coordination. The patients' rhythmic splits are involun-tary, unrelated to self or will or purpose. They hold the person at their mercy. His body is beset by meaningless tics, grimaces, spasms, jerks—every manner of rhythmic disturbance. Further-more, our artist of coordination is hired to split his rhythmic action for, say, twenty minutes. After a brilliant finale of "unified frag-mentation" he exits, and with rhythmic singleness of purpose, goes out for a bracing beer. But the patients are not so fortunate; the curtain never falls on their performances. Their sudden hand-claps, or foot-stamps, or elbow-poking, or knee-bouncings, or head-swivellings, or mouth-gapings take place at regular inter-vals. The strangely timed walks, the positions of prayer, the hasty searching through pages of an invisible book—hundreds of actions and combinations of movements—are relentlessly repeated. Whatever communication may be hidden behind them, such movements and the pauses between them recur in a definite rhythmical pattern. They possess the body that houses them. How can exorcise the demon of compulsion?

# *Agnes*

I've often wondered about the compulsive pattern of the rocking patients. Why do they do it? What feeling lies behind that rhythmical back-and-forth center massaging movement . . . ?

I sit down on the floor opposite the patient who rocks. She is listed on the charts as Agnes Porter, a label that has ceased to have any meaning for the human it designates. As exactly as possible, I adjust my legs to match hers: knees pulled up toward the body, feet about eighteen inches apart, only the heels in contact with the floor. The upper part of Agnes is more difficult for my body to imitate. Her chest is concave, her shoulders high and hunched with her head trapped between them. How strangely —like sticks—those arms poke out of the shoulder girdle. How limply the hands dangle from the wrist joints. How slackly the jaw hangs in that lackluster face, the lips lined with the white froth of medication. I force Agnes's position on my own body and try to enter her rocking pattern. How uncomfortably foreign it feels, alien to my own quality and tension. What enormous energy it takes to keep up with that fast, staccato tempo. The emphatic forward thrust of her movement creates in me a sensation of . . . fury? . . . defiance? . . . certainly of desperation. I feel caught, cramped, miserable; I don't like it at all. On and on and on we rock. . . . I'm getting slightly drowsy. . . . Strange, but there's something compellingly satisfying about this movement, after all. Doesn't the body's rhythmical back-and-forth movement over the genital area create an enjoyable sensation? Is this self-stimulation at the same time reassuring? Does it somehow enable Agnes to feel included in the fundamental purpose of existence? On and on and on we rock. . . . I'm aware that my body has gradually returned to its own softer tension, its own slower rhythm; my shoulders have relaxed. On and on and on I rock or sway or rotate, over and around the pivot of my pelvis. How comforting, how soothing . . . I think of all the mothers in this world since time began, cradling their babies in their arms, lulling them to sleep. Does Agnes's body seek to recapture the security and sensual warmth of this experience? Does her fierce seesawing quiet unbearable emotions, lull them to sleep? Does the rocking forestall a crisis? Back and forth, back and forth . . . I recall a time when my body mourned, in just this way, the death of one I loved. And I remember, too, that while it rocked and swayed and circled and cried, "I grieve," in the same breath it whispered, "I recover!"

During the hours and hours we rocked together, many more associations surfaced. Perhaps none of them applied to Agnes herself, but still . . . I somehow felt that I'd been temporarily a part of her world, and could begin to understand the need that lies behind the rocking action.

Sometimes, when I think of those of us in the world who are supposed to be normal, I'm astonished by the methods we use to counteract our fears. We ward off the "evil eye" with symbolic body signals: we cross our fingers, knock on wood, spit over our right (or left) shoulders. Woe betide the thespian who dares to whistle in the dressing room on opening night; he'll be responsible for the critics destroying the show if he doesn't step outside the door, spit, and turn around three times. How often have you gone back home for a forgotten object, and painstakingly sat down facing east and counted to ten before venturing forth under the cloud of the gods' hostility? Minutely detailed, accurately timed, and fantastically inventive are the human appeasement rites. No matter if these acts are senseless and time consuming, they assuage our guilts and our fears. We *have* to do them.

We're fortunate, however: we only indulge in such behavioral antics when confronted by the symbolic events that provoke them. Once the rituals are performed, that's that; we're safe again. The gods don't threaten us constantly. But the patients must repeat their routines of atonement over and over again in an endless attempt to stay the Punishing Hand.

As I enter the patient's compulsive action, I combine my

efforts with his in order to appease his controlling "demon." When it finally occurs to the patient that I am *with* him in the repetition of his movement, he begins to feel that I accept it, and therefore him. At that point, I start to make small variations, slight extensions from the original. I may speed the action up a bit, embellish it, simplify it. I may try to change the time lapses between the procedures, reassuring him that he can feel free to return to his own pattern whenever he must. This permission seems to take a load off his shoulders, and often reduces the frequency of the compulsive attacks. His need for the pattern is still being reinforced, and his right to perform it acknowledged. When the patient is able to change his compulsive appeasement motions, and comes to realize that nothing happens—absolutely nothing, no punishment, no disaster—then he has reached a turning point. With his approval, I can then begin to extend the changes further and further, and finally alter the pattern so strongly that neither he nor I nor the "One for whom he performed" can recognize the original pattern.

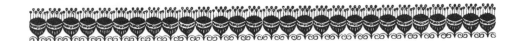

# SPACE
## Conquering the Void

Into the waiting emptiness of the great stage, the dancer's body soars in a breathtaking leap. Instantly, space acquires meaning and focus, as it converges on that arching form. Space is the dancer's domain, created just for him to fill with his joyous movement. He populates space with himself, extending his personality into its every level and direction. His body paints his images and fantasies upon its generous canvas.

In infancy, we view space from "underneath." Faces and objects loom large in our limited world. Are those great images comforting or frightening? A little later, space takes on another dimension as we toddle around amid the giants. Are we free to explore our fascinating new space-range in our own way, in our own time? Then comes the time of space-enchantment: trees to climb, sidewalks to run over, grass to be rolled on. Is our longing to consume space satisfied, or is there a frustrating ban on these joys? And finally we have become the "giants" ourselves, able

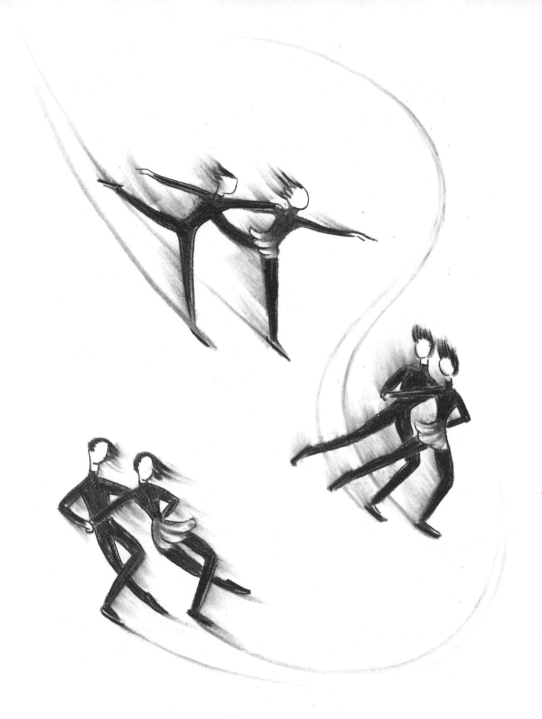

to comprehend the complete perspective of the space that surrounds us. How do we feel about it now?

Space can be experienced as an affliction as well as a gift. Our reactions to the height, depth, openness, or closed-ness of space can range from delight to out-and-out terror. A ride on a ski lift may be one man's rapture and another man's nightmare. A walk through Carlsbad Caverns can be fascinating or terrifying. Crowded elevators and subways, the vast, empty horizons of deserts and oceans, all evoke a diversity of individual reactions.

Space conditions seem to affect the characteristic behavior of whole nations. The awesome grandeur of the Alps that barricade my native Switzerland can't help but have a sobering influence on our nature. It's as if we were afraid of any vehement action or any daring thought which might disturb those "mountain gods" that watch over us. I know that we're regarded as inhibited, closed-in people, and our withheld body-expression supports that view. Our neighbors under the spacious, sunny skies of Italy, however, talk and gesture with emotional and physical abandon. We think of them as temperamental wine makers. They think of us as stingy innkeepers!

Man has always been actively involved in changing the appearance of his space: adding, cutting, shifting, rearranging his spatial environment for either practical or esthetic reasons. His concern over placement of things in space is reflected in the way he plans his garden and the way he decorates his home, clear down to the organization of his closets and bureau drawers. Man's bridges span his waters; his skyscrapers fragment his horizons; his freeways snake over the far reaches of his land.

With intricate calculations, we order the spatial relationships of other human beings. With careful consideration, we design our own weddings as well as our own funerals. Social, court, and military pageants are masterpieces in the art of body-placement. And how magnificently the Catholic Church choreographs its rites!

**Skaters encountering the void**

How generous is your "NO TRESPASSING" area which wards off the intrusion of other human bodies? How close can a loved one come to your person? A family member? A stranger? At what point do you begin to feel uneasy, and start to back away?

127

Or are you one who reserves no private space-territory?—one who can never get close enough, reaching out to all mankind with a touch, a pat, or a hug?

Many years ago, in the village of Kreuzlingen, there was a man who used to walk the streets, clinging so close to the fences and walls that I could hear his clothes brushing against them. We children, frightened but curious, would follow him at a distance. It was my first encounter with "crazy" space behavior.

Since then, I have seen many men and women, outside as well as inside hospitals, moving along as if shying away from something that might be lying in wait ahead of them. And there are so many other disturbances that I see clearly performed in space:

> Bodies that look flattened out, progressing sideways as if between two walls.
> Bodies bumping into other bodies, and bodies that wind carefully around bodies that aren't there.
> Bodies weighted down by invisible burdens, and bodies carried as if gazing into rosy-tinted skies.
> Bodies sneaking around like legacy hunters.
> Bodies cowering as if entering a burning building.

I see apology designed into space, and degradation, and lowness, and meanness. . . . But most of all, I see fear engraved on these bodies; space has become the enemy.

Instead of passively being invaded by space, the patients must learn to become the invaders. In the sessions, we declare war against the threat of space. The patients line up against the wall. With arms linked to form an invincible human chain, the line of battle charges into the danger zone. Step by step, gaining territory as we pass through the menacing vacuum, we attack space as if it were tangible. Punching, kicking, poking, we leap over it, jump on it, cut through it, crawl under it, and heave it out of the way. As action replaces passivity, space—a vanquished element—loses its terrors.

**Fear of space**

The way a body uses space can provide specific information about the individual who owns it. Does a body know where it stands in space? (Has the person a definite point of view?)

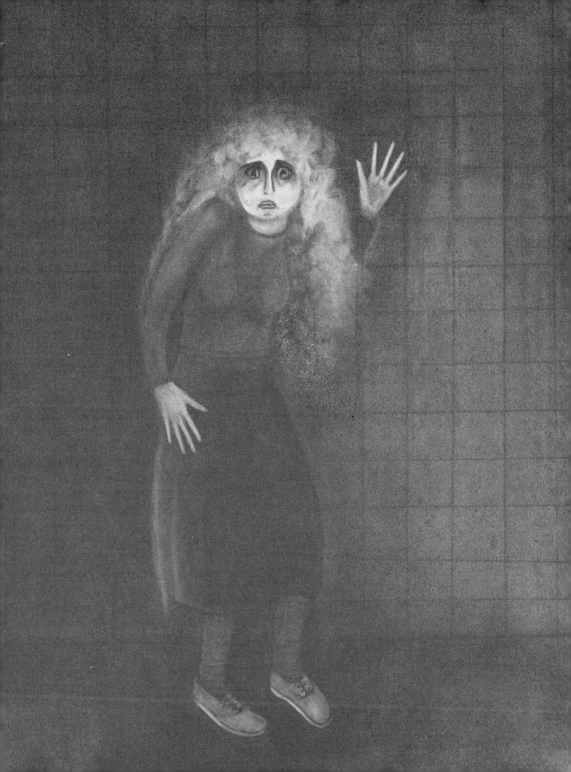

Can a body maintain a directional course? (Is the person a man of conviction?) Is the whole body unified in the effort to change direction in space? (Can the person make decisions?) Can the body confront, straight-on, the other bodies that share his space? (Can the person face reality?)

I apply every means available to create targets for confrontation, teaching the bodies to "stand their ground," the eyes to look steadily and "take in," the individuals to "level" with one another.

# Henry

For three years, I worked in a hospital with a more open setting, where the patients were more reachable and the atmosphere less confining. One morning, I decided to do a study in partners, which required one of them to give space-commands for the other to obey. With simple gestures, the leader was to tell his follower to come, go, sit, jump up, run, change direction, go over to that corner, turn around, and so forth. When one partner had acted as the boss for quite a while, the other would take the lead. I figured that it would be a satisfying experience for the patients to tell somebody else what to do and how to behave, it being the reverse of any feelings they might have about being pushed around. And it might lead to some brand-new space actions.

The exercise worked out fine for most of the patients; they had a great time thinking up movement tasks for their partners. If one person became too bossy, I encouraged his partner to refuse to obey or, better still, to start giving orders himself. A healthy self-assertion built up in most of them, and the feeling of power made them think up commanding gestures, strong enough and pertinent enough to be easily followed.

Not so with one couple. It was the woman who conducted the action at all times; the man eagerly fulfilled her wishes, never once venturing to disobey, or give a command to her.

"Why don't you tell Hilda what to do for a change?" I asked at last.

Henry smiled at me helplessly, and after attempting a few

assertive movements, which looked more like desperate requests for Hilda's compliance, said apologetically:

"It's no use; I'm like this. At home, my wife tells me what to do: 'Go and take the cans out; go and bring the cans in; put the sprinklers on; don't forget to bring some money home; you need a haircut; we're going to the Chandler's tonight, so don't forget to shave!' Trudi, I just can't do this exercise!"

"Will you try it once with me, Henry?" I asked. "I'd like to obey you for a while. You only have to make big, clear signals so I'll know for sure what you want me to do."

His commands were very vague at first; I really had to guess what they meant. But I turned around, sat down, jumped up, following them as best I could. He couldn't believe his eyes. It must have seemed so easy all of a sudden, for his courage grew. He began to enjoy bossing me around—thoroughly! His gestures took on the authority of an emperor; they were emblazoned on space. And they sent me into a frenzy of activity. I ran, I turned somersaults, I bent over double; I fell, I crawled, and I leapt, until I collapsed exhausted into a chair. We both laughed, and Henry threw his arms around me in a hug.

I didn't see him around the next day, but I really hadn't expected him to show up for the session after his abrupt change from putty-man to dictator. It took Henry almost a week to recover from his "trip." When he did return, his manner was subdued, but there was a new glint in his eye. He began to work with unaccustomed concentration. Of course, there were setbacks, but the initial grain of self-determination had been implanted in his mind. His movements gradually gained confidence, and the give and take with his dance partners began to show that he could clearly state his needs.

The day Henry left the hospital, he introduced me to his wife, a tiny, smiling woman with a pointed nose that looked as if it could peck. Behind her back, Henry winked at me and made a comical gesture in her direction, as if to say, "From now on, girl, it's going to be a fifty-fifty proposition!"

Parallel to a person's inability to "face" certain things, exists his tendency to evade, to hide his person as well as his feelings. Since most of my patients have been hiding for years behind their masks and delusions, I try very hard to bring whatever is concealed out into the open. I first ask them to hide their faces, their hands, their chests, their pelvises from the view of any outsider. Since they are all masters at the art of concealment, there's not much change in their appearances. Some seem pleased to hide parts of themselves they'd never thought about hiding before—elbows and toes, for example. Eventually, though, I want those bodies to emerge, to participate in the freedom of space.

So the studio becomes a huge arena, surrounded by grandstands. I choose this particular space facility because there's simply no place to hide in it; within its vast circumference, a person is completely exposed on all sides. What's more, the idea of the arena is loaded with images from which the patients can draw: the politician, the bull fighter, the fire-and-brimstone preacher, the fashion model—any person who not only wants to be looked at, but *must* be looked at. One by one, the patients walk around the ring. Here comes the "King," proudly displaying the head that wears the crown. And here is a runner, bearing aloft a flaming torch for the world to see. And this is the "General," exhibiting the medals on his puffed-out chest. Every person thus imagines a reason for showing off some part of his body.

When our arena becomes the background for a circus, the patients are imitating performers whose success *depends* on their ability to project themselves. In a real circus, there is no doubt who is who, and to which act each one of them belongs. With spacious gestures they indicate their forthcoming feats. Each movement is precisely drawn for instant communication. Each one of these circus performers dominates the immense space with his body. The intensity of his focus exacts the focus of his onlookers; his whole body demands the attention on which it thrives.

The patients may start out uncertainly, tentatively. But slowly the roles take over, and lion tamers, clowns, tightrope walkers, and acrobats begin to emerge. I see the individuals moving in space in ways they've never shown me before, directing themselves toward a single purpose with new focus and concentration. I see them developing new spatial relationships with one another; and for the first time, their gestures begin to take on the directness of communication demanded by the roles they play.

I try insofar as is possible to segregate the elements of movement, even though each element is an inseparable part of the whole. But I feel that focusing on one area or another can give form and purpose to a session, and at the same time establish that area more conclusively in the patient's awareness. This method (if it can be called a method) affords a definite course for me to follow as I work my way through the intricate mazes of schizophrenic disturbances.

All I know is that this approach seems to guarantee contact with the individual, almost without exception. It insures reaction; any patient I've ever worked with has responded in some way, has shown himself differently. And every response is a vital source of information. How often I've wished for the presence of the ward psychiatrist when a patient suddenly changes his movement pattern, or displays an uncharacteristic feeling-reaction, or begins, unexpectedly, to verbalize. There's no doubt that dance therapy can offer new body-experiences, which in turn can engender new mind-experiences, thus furnishing new material for psychiatric examination.

There was a time when I was concerned with the scientific investigation of movement. I wanted to research, to categorize, to measure, rate, and bundle up neatly the resulting statistics. But after a time I realized that I had neither the academic background nor the mathematical nature to pursue such a monumental undertaking. Some day, perhaps, therapists will be able to calculate in degrees the physical manifestation of emotion, and devise an exact psychological translation of movement. Until that time, I, at least, will rely on the expression of the body. I will act upon what I see.

In the course of my own experience, I have created an imaginary "model therapist" on whom to base my behavior. Here is the ideal I conceived.

She is:

> flexible without being irresolute
> definite without being authoritative
> warm without being sentimental
> imaginative without being frivolous

sensitive to needs of others without over-identification

intuitive and spontaneous within the realistic framework of her objective.

She possesses:

an affectionate respect for mankind in general

the ability to refrain from moral judgments

the ability to differentiate between functional and nonfunctional body postures and movements

a body that can demonstrate whatever she is trying to teach

the ability to cope with any negative aspect of her own nature.

Every therapist evolves, through experience, her own way of working. I have found that a certain amount of structure helps me to organize my ideas. Whatever theme I have chosen to present runs through a session like a thread, binding consecutive portions together. This kind of reinforcement gives the members of my class a sense of security, of having familiar ground under their feet.

# Basic structure

IDEA: Working with contrasting extremes

1. *Theme:* A malfunction of any aspect of the body

   a. Physical representation of the manfunction (how is it exhibited in the body?)

   b. Psychological representation of the malfunction (what feelings can be associated with this body?)

   c. Physical and psychological representations of the malfunction's opposite extreme

   d. Working device (correction of the malfunction through exposure to its contrasting extreme)

2. *Warm-up*

   a. Registering the mood presented by the group, and adapting or adjusting the session accordingly, working to keep it easy-going and non-threatening

   b. Personal introductions (using names, movement, rhythms, breathing, and sounds)

   c. Group contact (interaction in various ways)

3. *Instruction:* Exercises which increase the body's functional possibilities, while at the same time preparing the body for expression of whatever contrast you have chosen

   a. On floor or standing in place (any dancer's exercises for establishing adequate breathing, strengthening muscles, correcting distortions, and, in general, extending the body's vocabulary)

   b. In space (walks, runs, jumps, hops, leaps, skips, turns—any and all of which movements can be combined in various ways and extended immeasurably by the application of specific rhythms, tensions, qualities, and space patterns)

4. *Expression:* Connecting the basic theme to life situations

   a. Allowing the patient's body to experience fully his ineffectual position in life

   b. Allowing the patient's body to experience fully the contrasting state of being

5. *Creating the functional balance between the two aspects of the theme:* Changing the energy level of both extremes, until the body approximates physical and emotional balance

6. *Conclusion:* In any movement form, reinforce pleasurably the two aspects of the theme with which you have been working during the particular session, always trying to leave the patient in a state of well-being.

SAMPLE SESSION I

IDEA: Working with contrasting extremes

1. *Theme* (a malfunction): The passive body

   a. Physical representations of the malfunction: loose tension, slow breathing, inward focus, minimum movement, lethargy, sluggish reactions

b. Psychological representations of the malfunction: apathy, indifference, depression, exhaustion, despair, detachment

c. Physical and psychological representations of the opposite extreme (the overactive body): hyperactive movements, dynamic energy, outward focus, highly animated expression, intense overinvolvement

d. Working device: Activating the passive body through exposure to overactivity

2. *Warm-up:* Begin to present qualities associated with passivity and activity

a, b, and c: Use slow and fast, strong and soft, tight and loose, in movement, breathing, and sound.

3. *Instruction:* In all exercises, encourage the body toward animated activity; prepare it for expression.

a and b: Mobilize body parts; mobilize the whole body.

Focus attention on self, on others, on various points in space, making sure the entire being is involved in the focus.

Focus the whole body into a chosen direction (use specific floor patterns: squares, circles, trangles, zigzags).

Include centering exercises, sound, and breathing.

Increase energy in all elements of movement.

4. *Expression:* Connect the passive body, and then the overactive body, to life situations.

a. Ask: "What kind of people behave this way?" (Typical answers: lazy, bored, shy, depressed.) Have the class enact these ultra-passive characters, clearly emphasizing the body's behavior in each case: its tempo, alignment, use of space . . .

b. Ask: "What kind of people are constantly rushing and dashing around?" (Typical answers: nervous, pressured, bossy, nosy.) Now enact these characters, again pointing out the body's behavior.

5. *Creating a balance*

   To a given rhythm, alternate the unfunctional extremes of the overactive and the too passive.

   Now, alternate the functional aspects of active and passive (focussed, direct movement, and then calm, relaxed movement).

6. *Conclusion:* Positive reinforcement

   Using any simple form and rhythm, begin by having members of the class move about as a group with strong, out-going bodies, contacting one another. Alternate this with inward focus, represented by calm, relaxed movements.


SAMPLE SESSION II

IDEA: Working with a prevailing affect

1. *Theme:* The fearful body (contrast: the coping body)
   a. Physical representations of the fearful body: retreat, helplessness, contraction, shaking, irregular breathing
   b. Psychological representations of the fearful body: inability to face life, seek new experiences, relate effectively, or cope with emergencies; feeling of isolation, helplessness
   c. Physical and psychological representations of the coping body: expanded movement, centeredness and flexibility, strong tension, deep, regular breathing, confidence, eagerness, ability to face life's challenges
   d. Working device: Releasing the body from fear through use of effective methods of coping

2. *Warm-up:* As indicated in BASIC STRUCTURE, in this case emphasizing centered body and various degrees of tension.

3. *Instruction*

   In all exercises—on floor, standing in place, or moving in space—work to promote physical representations of a fearless body.

Contrast the above with physical representations of a fearful body.

(Note: in each case, avoid using the descriptive word "fearless.")

4. *Expression*

Ask: "When does your body act this way?" (Typical answer: "When I'm scared.")

Ask: "What are you scared of?" (Typical answers include snakes, height, doorknobs, violence, the unknown, the dark, death, noises, being alone, people.)

Ask: "What do you do when you're afraid?" (Some will suggest hide, run, collapse, scream, freeze up. Others will offer, "Fight him!" "Scare him worse than he scares me." "Face it— really look and find out what's there.")

Now perform every one of these fear reactions.

a and b: Perform first the helpless reactions, then the heedlessly aggressive reactions, in both cases trying to create full physical and emotional involvement.

5. *Creating a balance*

To a given rhythm, alternate the unfunctional extremes of helpless panic and blind aggression.

Now, emphasizing the positive value that can be found within each of these reaction types, change the energy levels of each, to achieve gradually the functional balance between active confrontation and intelligent retreat.

6. *Conclusion:* Making the necessary adjustments in breathing and tension, create control over the prevailing affect by translating fear and attack into harmonious movement forms.

*Note:* This session should be followed by a session dealing with realistic fear vs. unrealistic fear.

The reason for working with the extremes of any emotion or physical state is that they are so easy for anyone to comprehend. Once the extremes have been established, we can work with the many and varied degrees that exist between them.

Any reactions are valuable assets to a session. They open to the patients new areas of experience and increase the therapist's store of information. The therapist should always try to use the individual reaction, rather than ignoring it in favor of a reaction with which she is more familiar.

The outlines I've presented are planning ideas, and certainly must not be thought of as binding. The therapist must be free and able at any time to deviate from her original working ideas whenever the patients' moods or reactions take another tangent.

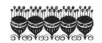

# Part 3

# BETWEEN TWO WORLDS

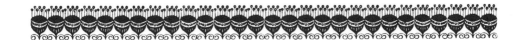

# IMPROVISATION AND FORMULATION

## Making Friends with Dragons

As he has participated in the elements of dance, the patient has become better acquainted with his physical being. His movements show signs of being more facile, functional, and appropriate. Also, his body has experienced many commonplace forms of emotional expression, a sort of movement vocabulary with which to register his own feelings. Now he can be led much further along the road to the *understanding* of his feeling self. He is ready for improvisation.

Improvisation is a form of "physical doodling," a process of non-verbal free association during which the individual permits his body to move spontaneously and unguardedly. Elimination of the mind's controlling influence can cause underlying feelings, long rooted in the subconscious, to erupt into the body. Their actual physical performance brings them into the person's subjective awareness. It can be a stunning experience to find your body suddenly acting out a long-repressed sorrow, a hidden fury, an unacknowledged fear, or an inhibited sex drive. In such movement breakthroughs, your body is telling you about feelings you didn't know you had. And there's no denying the authenticity of those feelings.

After living through such a penetrating experience, a person is emotionally spent for the time being. He attains a temporary neutral vantage point from which he can view himself dispassionately, and contrast the violence of his newly exposed feeling-expression with his actual present reality. Recognition of the disparity between the two can lead to further self-evaluation and a conscious wish for change.

As I try to put this whole theory into practice, my first undertaking is to restore the person's body-freedom, the freedom he lost when his mind began to censor his body's behavior. But it's not so easy to turn off that mental editing machinery. How can I get his body to act on its own, his mind not to think?

I ask the individual to assume any comfortable position and direct his attention back into his body, to sense his heartbeat, his breathing, his entire physical self. Then I suggest that he permit his body to change its behavior, whenever and however it needs to do so. Long intervals of waiting may follow these directions, but sooner or later the body will begin to move. And surprisingly enough, it will move in ways that it has not moved before.

The longer a body can stand the absence of mental control, the more its feelings will be set free and become displayed in the very movement that engendered them. In this way, it comes about that a person suddenly hears his body crying, sees his body hitting, feels his body falling or running . . . running. In these physical expressions of his feelings, the person confronts himself. He catches himself in the act.

This experience is never disagreeable, no matter how the body has behaved. On the contrary, it's exciting to learn that there's more to you than you've ever recognized. But there's a more significant reason for the sense of well-being that follows such an episode. Whatever feeling comes into the body, the individual finds himself expressing it without conflict. For once, he has given himself the right to luxuriate in the total acting-out of an emotion.

# *Lily*

At age twenty-four, Lily looked fourteen and behaved like a baby. Extreme disturbance was written all over her. Her stockings were crumpled down over her child-like, shapeless legs; her blouse was held together by its last remaining button. Matted hair covered her forehead and eyes, and the dirty doll that she always had with her dangled from one hand, or was squeezed under her armpit. Lily's communication amounted to two expressions: one of wanting, the other of not wanting. Her begging was supported by the only two words that ever came out of her mouth: "Say yes!" Her denials were vocalized in long, foghorn-like sounds.

Lily was in one of the afternoon classes, and every morning I worked with her alone. At first, there was no way at all to structure our private sessions. I followed her in anything she would initiate, which was usually very little. But sometimes she would run a bit and smile, or skip a bit and smile. These activities were frequently interrupted by visits to the bathroom. She would sit on the seat, completely dressed, and soak herself thoroughly. At the same time, she would pull her right breast out of her blouse and suck on it. After a while, she'd stuff it back into her blouse and stand up. I'd try to clean her up somehow, washing off her hands and legs; and all the while Lily made soft purring sounds of baby-like tenderness.

One afternoon in Lily's class, I asked the patients to walk about the room however they wanted to walk, but if they found that their bodies wanted to move some other way, to go ahead and let them. For a long, long time everybody walked around the hall. Then one became faster, another one slower. Somebody began to flap his arms. Somebody else began to spin around. This one sat down; that one lay down. There was a sound of crying and a sound of laughing. Lily still plodded on, her face expressionless as if in a trance. Suddenly she screamed, turned, and dashed over to fling her arms around me, shrieking, "I'm afraid, I'm afraid! *I want my Mommy!*" I held her until her screaming stopped, then took her hand in a firm grip and walked her briskly around the room. Gradually she quieted down. . . . And tomorrow we could continue where we left off today.

Though Lily's infantile state had long been apparent, on this day her body had regenerated the immediacy of her emotional need. And Lily had communicated that need in a normal outburst, realistically performed and appropriately verbalized.

Once a person's feelings of conflict have been brought into the body, improvisation has served its main purpose. There's no point in going on and on with it, for no matter how many times the body "admits" to a feeling, it will continue to express it in the same manner, over and over. Though the surplus of energy and of affect will be temporarily discharged, it will only accumulate again . . . to be discharged again . . . to accumulate again. . . . It can become a mindless circle, a kind of self-indulgence. There will be no change in the problem itself. Something constructive has to be done about it.

The time has come for the individual to present his subjective, free-floating feeling in an objective, explicit form, with his body as the instrument for his composition. This production requires him to organize the forces of both his mind and his body as he does something about himself, with himself. As he develops a logical framework for his expression, seeks movement patterns for it, gives it a particular rhythm, a certain step, a special tension, he is gaining the upper hand. He is disciplining the feeling which has, up to now, held him at its mercy. His completed production has two positive results: he is now able to experience that feeling without conflict, and he can communicate it accurately and realistically. Other people can recognize it. They can react to it. And their response reinforces his own identity.

Patients have chosen many, many dance forms to show me their feelings, their conflicts, their confusions, their fantasies. Hate was clarified by the rhythm of a tango. Its movements began with the little stamps, followed by brusque turns, lashing arms, and ending in a crouched, threatening position. Loneliness was demonstrated by a patient walking in an inward spiral; its reduc-

146

ing circumference shut out more and more of the world around him, until he stood still at its center, wrapped in isolation. The sensation of being lost was once depicted by a patient using searching movements, running from one direction to another, turning in confusion, and hopelessly hunting for a way out. This woman's desperation was suddenly resolved by the spontaneous reaction of another patient, who had been watching intently. With matter-of-fact directness, she walked over to the lost individual and led her in a straight line out of her dilemma and into a chair.

# *Alice*

When I first met Alice, she was sitting in the hospital studio, shaken and crying.

"They want to separate me from my friends on Venus," she sobbed. "They told me that's what they want to do! They said that's why they give me shock treatments!"

During my sessions in the following weeks, Alice often talked about her "sweet friends, far up there."

"How would it be, Alice," I asked one day, "if you would tell all of us here in the group how your friends look and what they do that makes you love them so much?"

"Well . . . ," she began hesitantly, "they're all so happy to see me when I come up to them. And sometimes Clandestine gives me a kiss."

Nobody in the group had to be told what to do. Awkwardly but with affection, they shook Alice's hand. They patted her. They smiled. Their greetings must have pleased her, because she continued her description.

"They lie on golden couches . . . they drink out of golden goblets . . . they fly all around on their golden wings. They have golden dragons—very friendly ones—to play with and ride on." And Alice began to teach her willing cast how these beautiful people moved and flew and drank and played.

"But there's always the chimes . . . the lovely wind-music . . . and I've never heard that here."

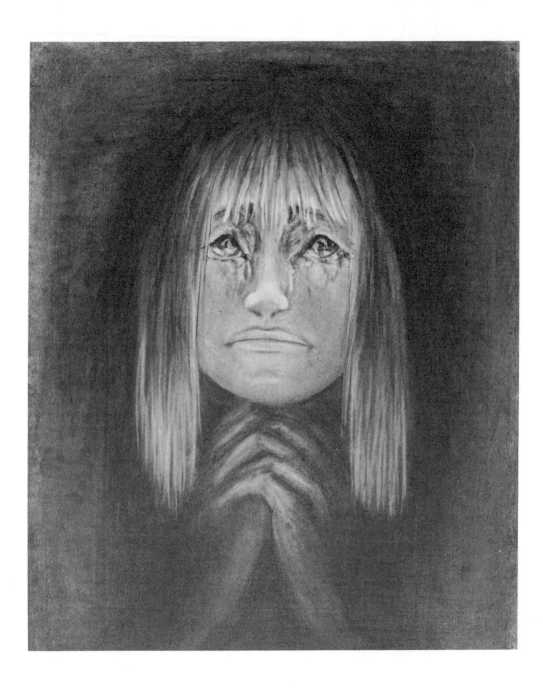

148

I brought out my bells and triangle and gong. Soon the room was filled with delightfully eerie sounds. It all ended in a floating, flying sort of dance, with everyone trying his best to be courteous and friendly—and golden! Rarely have I seen a stage director directing his group so convincingly, or performers who could so easily identify with his images.

Alice provided a lovely fantasy for us to follow, but there have also been terrifying ones: monsters with hideous faces, a fierce tiger whose long tail writhed in weird geometrical designs, an infuriated god with crimson eyes, a group of sinister black-hooded figures armed with gleaming knives. I was shown how frighteningly these visions moved, how threateningly they spoke, and even heard about the terrible things they commanded their subjects to do.

Whatever the content of a patient's delusion, whatever its psychological origins, its enactment brings about three valid results:

1. He has been enabled to share the secrecy of his delusion, to expose it and to cope with it; he has destroyed its power to control his existence.
2. Both sides of a person's existence have been recognized, and he can contrast reality with delusion. Alice knew, in the session that day, that she was in the hospital studio, not on Venus, and that the one who kissed her was good old Betty, not Clandestine. But weren't these earth people responding to her in much the same way as her planetary friends? Perhaps it would not be so necessary to take refuge on that other planet. Perhaps reality was not so bad after all!
3. Because the physical production of a person's imaginary world requires constant evaluation of both sides, he is led toward the discovery of the healthy balance between fantasy and reality.

Alice

Don't artists go through the exact same process? Don't they move easily between two worlds as they realize a flight of fancy in a poem, a symphony, a sculpture, a dance? We wouldn't want to try to stop the artist from seeing or hearing his fantastic

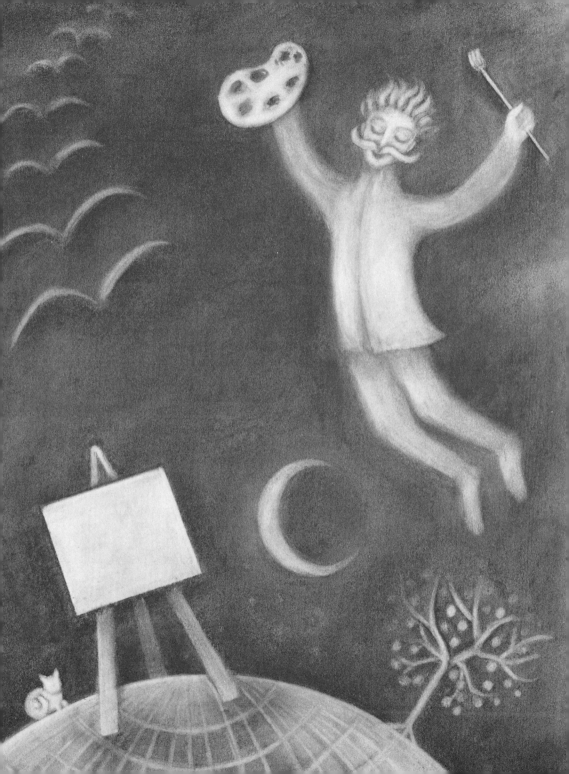

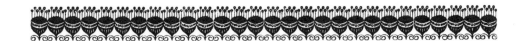

# DANCE

## Is Dance <u>Really</u> Therapeutic?

"If you feel that dance is so therapeutic, how come a great dancer like Nijinsky went crazy?" So goes the question of dance therapy skeptics. It can be answered, I think, by the fact that ballet is not specifically designed to influence the dancer's mind. As a performing art, it demands a highly specialized technique, which is evolved into an exquisitely realized style. Years and years of dedicated practice, of unremitting self-discipline, are required to master its intricate forms and patterns. The dancer can only express his individuality within the confines of these set configurations. It must have been constantly necessary for Nijinsky to suppress his emotional conflicts in order to achieve his incredible technical skill. A life of training and performing must have allowed him precious little opportunity to show who he *really* was or what he was *really* feeling. Three *tours en l'air*, brilliantly executed, could never provide a release from his anxieties or a solution to his personal problems. They could, and did, display the miraculous mastery he had over his own body. In a controlling society, he mastered a controlling technique. He had to deny "the human" in order to become "the dancer."

My "dancers" are exposed only to the technical requirements necessary to heighten the body's functionality. The only "style" they learn is represented by my concept of the ideal body. Within their own limitations, they try to achieve the highest physical level of all the movements common to man. They aren't concerned with any preconceived dance combinations. They create their own forms to express their own feelings. Each individual makes his own uniquely personal statement—emotionally as well as motionally.

It has been fascinating when from time to time I've worked with dancer-patients. Their emotional disturbances may be more difficult to detect at first, simply because they move more skillfully, coordinate better, extend more impressively, and in general use their bodies more artistically than the average person. But upon closer observation, I've discovered that this very same technical prowess can become a perfect facade, an ideal defense behind which a person's disturbance can be safely hidden.

# Hanna

Hanna was referred to me by a psychiatrist for private sessions at my studio. A lovely girl, highly trained in modern dance, she moved in an exquisitely fluid, formalized style. She looked like a goddess—serene, detached, far above and beyond either good or bad—and she described with her body exactly that. I knew that I must bring the lonely goddess back to earth, to enable her to express conflict as well as harmony, to trust her own feelings; in short, to return her to her own reality.

As I worked with Hanna, I saw that she designed a kind of magic circle around herself, remaining isolated within its limits. Nothing, or no one, could encroach upon the boundaries of this circle, nor was there any possibility for her to reach out beyond it. Her hands were always in a rejecting position: flexed, creating a sharp stop in relation to her arms. Her center was consistently contracted, permitting no extension of herself. Certainly no personal feeling ever erupted within the circular form she designed. Totally noncommittal, her movements were beautifully boring to watch.

I had to bring that talented body into a position from which two-way communication could be established. I had to change the flexed angle of her hands so that they could reach out and draw in. I wanted to loosen up the reserved chest and pelvis, to release the immovable center, and to tear down the unfunctional defense that was symbolized by that miserable circle. Hanna had a hard time relinquishing all of her protective measures. She talked; she struggled; she cried; but I remained adamant in my belief that I'd have to change her body's behavior in order to change its feeling content.

During a long period of improvisation, Hanna began to destroy her old image. The time came when she finally managed to rip away the arty forms, the virtuoso techniques, to see what reality lay underneath. When she finally began to give shape to the ugly parts of her feelings, the dances she composed were original and expressive. Distortion and dissonance were now a part of her range, contrasting with the harmony to give her movements a new depth. Now Hanna was free to present every facet of her nature to the world. She no longer had to hide behind a technique that was alien to her true feelings. She had created a much more fascinating form which enabled her to use them. Her compositions were now true statements of emotion, and as such were satisfying to the dancer, and compelling for the onlooker. The goddess had descended from her pedestal and become human.

# George

About a year later, another dancer was referred to me. George's mode of expression was different from Hanna's; in fact, it was quite the opposite. Instead of hiding behind a form, he used his technical skill to exhibit his conflicts *fully*. His body endlessly repeated the same movements. It pulled in all directions at once, every which way: staccato, jerky, cramped, and at all times in high gear. Involved in panicky convulsions of movement, he seemed to tear himself to pieces, leaving his mutilated body parts scattered all over the floor.

When George improvised in my class for the first time, the other members of the class spontaneously applauded. But then, as time went on, all of us could see that he responded to any theme I introduced with exactly the same executions. The group gradually began to lose interest in his performances, became resentful of them, and finally rejected dancer and man altogether. His repetition of the same subjective, sterile form was merely a compulsive mannerism, no matter how brilliantly it was presented.

Since I couldn't suppress George's need to display his conflict, I went right along with it, asking for stronger tension, faster tempo, more conflicting pulls, more combative distortions. I pressed him to the point where he could find out for himself how hopelessly he was stuck in the same movement groove. If I had insisted on an immediate change in the beginning, I would only have added another enemy to his list. As it was, I gave him the support he needed to confront the futility of his unrealistic opposition.

About this time, I assigned him a task. I asked him to choreograph his own dance. For weeks George worked by himself, enlisting the aid of only one fellow student for the quite complicated lighting and sound effects. I was the only guest invited to his premiere. He called his dance *Phantasmagoria*.

George's head appeared from beneath the curtain at floor level, center stage. This head's eyes were changing focus in a frantic staccato: Up! Down! Side! Down! Side! Up! Slowly the whole creature crawled forward, its body and limbs taking over the spastic movements that had begun with the eyes. While his fragmented body struggled to its feet, George found himself surrounded by giant shadows. Those phantasms of his own contorted self became his antagonists in a violent struggle, as he battled furiously for his own identity. He attacked those body-ghosts one by one. He shot them; he choked them; he clawed them to ribbons; he knocked them flat and trampled them to death . . . until not one of the specters remained. The whole scene was underscored by deafening electronic sounds, meant to symbolize the expiration of the monsters. As the monsters vanished, there came a great silence . . . an arrest in time . . . a cessation of experiencing. Into this stillness the beat of his heart emerged, pounding through the loudspeaker. Then the transformation began to take place. Calm and strength began to flow through his exhausted body. The drumming heartbeat quieted and became a softly pulsating melody. As he stood there, George's whole attitude reflected peace and concordance. He slowly turned and looked back at the scene of his conquest, secure in the knowledge that his phantasms, the symbols of his conflict, had been laid to rest. With a last, beautifully freeing gesture, George strode triumphantly toward a new life, as the curtain slowly fell.

George's involvement in this memorable production, and his concentration on the choreography of his problematic condition, directed his energy and real talent toward clear and effective communication. As he began to take constructive action to remove the distortions of his body, he also acted to resolve the conflicts of his life.

I've tried to introduce you to a few of the people who helped me as I struggled to find a way to help them. I'll always be grateful to them for verifying my belief in the healing value of dance. Throughout the years I've spent in their company, I tried to reach certain definite goals:

1. To identify for each person the specific parts of his body that have been unused or misused, and to direct his actions into functional patterns.
2. To establish the unifying interactive relationship between mind and body, between fantasy and reality.
3. To bring subjective emotional conflict into an objective physical form, where it can be perceived and dealt with constructively.
4. To use every aspect of movement that will increase the individual's ability to adapt adequately to his environment and to experience himself as a whole, functioning human being.

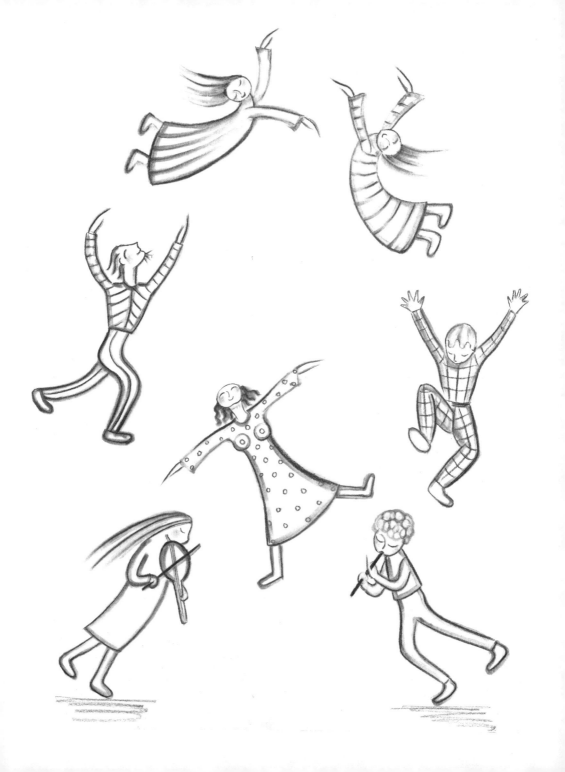

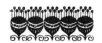

*Part 4*

*LUKE*

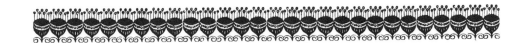

# THE METAMORPHOSIS OF A MANNERISM

## "Nobody Showed Me How to be a Man"

### The shape of fear

About a year after I had stopped working at the state hospital, I began, one day, to sort through my accumulated masses of notes. Among them was a well-worn chocolate-brown folder with the name "Luke" on its cover. Luke was a patient I had worked with for over a year on a one-to-one basis. The first page in the folder was a brief progress report that I'd written on his case:

> Patient was severely regressed at beginning of treatment. Deteriorated ego; little relationship to himself or to world around him. Physically weak and tense. Afraid to move. Distorted body image and strong mannerism. No verbalization.
> Affect: suspicious, fearful, apologetic. Early contact was made with therapist and continued throughout treatment. Patient became aware of mannerism; began to

163

talk about it, explain its meaning, and finally discontinued it altogether. Eventually, patient was able to express his real problems. Verbalized clearly. Showed a desire to draw; interest in sketching continued throughout. Personality developed slowly, but consistently. Changes were manifested in movement, in verbalizations, in drawings.

How bland it all sounded! What a cut-and-dried account of all those hours we'd struggled with each other. I remembered so clearly every detail of that first meeting. . . .

Alone in my studio one morning, I glanced up to see a black man standing in the doorway. I hadn't heard him arrive; when my eyes accidentally touched him I didn't know whether he was coming in or leaving. He just stood there, strangely weightless and ghost-like, wrapped in deep silence. Finally, carefully, he began to move, circling the room slowly, like a trapped animal. He kept very close to the walls, and his feet seemed to touch the floor only slightly, as if the touch hurt him. I sensed fear with him, all around him—but the feeling of fear itself seemed to have been burnt out of his body. All that remained was the shape of fear, a design of fear.

As I stood, fascinated, and watched Luke edge his way around the room, I became acquainted with his peculiar personal mannerism for the first time. It consisted of three distinct, separate actions, repeated one after the other, always in the same order. To begin, he would suddenly raise both arms in a sweeping arc, which ended with his hands forming precise, devil-like horns on his forehead. Maintaining this devilish or faun-like position, he would make a great, deep bow, then return to his standing posture. For the second movement he would flatten his hands, palms turned down and, using them as if they were sharp cutting instruments, make slicing gestures along his neck. In the final movement he would drop his head on his chest and stroke his hair forward with soft, tender strokes. These three meticulous motions, done in a definite rhythm and with a gentle grace, created an atmosphere of pious humility.

**Luke's mannerisms**

His mannerism fascinated me. Could it be an extremely devout greeting? And if so, whom does one have to greet so

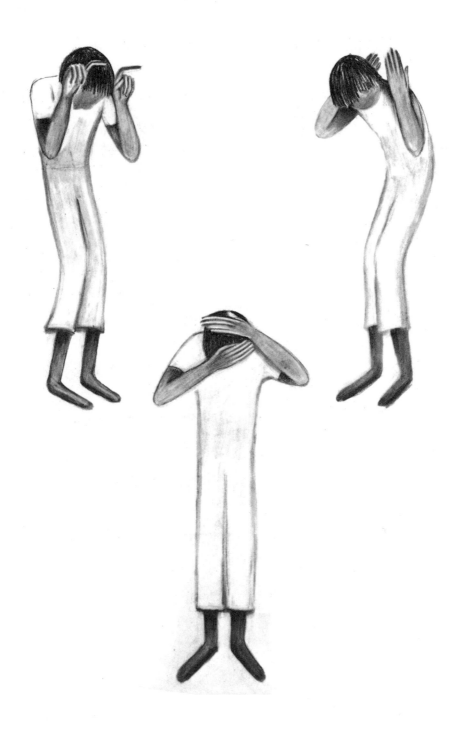

humbly, so frequently, and so elaborately? My curiosity about Luke was not to be satisfied in a hurry. There was very little I could do with him in the beginning, except to be there in the room and accompany him in his silent circling of the walls, observing his appearance and behavior. Luke's skin was a light café-au-lait color. He had a beautiful oval-shaped face, and limbs that were very long and fine; his hands were small and soft-looking. His eyes were always downcast—never focusing straight ahead and only occasionally darting quick glances to one side or the other. He kept his body in an extreme backward slant: chest caved in, back rounded, head forced down. He bounced when he walked, but it wasn't a happy bounce: the "down" was emphasized rather than the "up." His rigidly held torso rocked back and forth, so that his body looked as if it were saying, "Yes, yes, yes," over and over again. And always, always there were the horns, the cuttings, and the head pattings.

Little by little I tried to interrupt his walking and introduce other movements. He would respond to my suggestions by muttering, "Oh. Oh-oh," giving the one word every manner of inflection and connotation, like an actor searching for the best reading of a line.

"Will you jump with me, Luke, like this?"

"Oh. OH!" And he'd give a sort of hop-hop.

"That's good. Now can you jump with both feet at the same time?"

"Oh? Oh, oh, oh . . . ooh-ooh." And he would revert to his mannerism.

Luke seemed to have no knowledge of his body as a whole, and had trouble locating his body parts. He didn't always know where his head was, and if I asked him to touch his shoulders he would touch his elbows. His concentration span was extremely limited, and any new movement I suggested seemed to trigger his mannerism. He couldn't manage a skip, but he would run a bit, and learned to slide. When I asked him for a throwing motion, his hand would make a fist in the throw, and open up on the return. Luke cut off the air sharply when he inhaled, like a gasp, and could only release air in stingy amounts, keeping most of it stored up in his lungs. A tight tension prevailed over his body; he couldn't relax his muscles. He couldn't relax, period. He didn't know left from right, up from down, slow from fast. He wouldn't sit down or remove his shoes. He avoided being touched. And he wouldn't speak—except for his marvelous variety of "Oh, oh"s. All of Luke's non-doings were performed with such a self-effacing charm that it almost seemed a pity to interfere with his behavior.

Luke appeared to be fascinated by his hands. He would stretch them out and look at them in amazement, then contort his face into violent grimaces of loathing. I tried to encourage him to make different movements with his hands, but he'd only fall immediately back into his mannerism. One day, I reached out my hands toward him in a gesture of acceptance and friendship. He stared at my open palms for a long moment, then uttered his first clear statement of fact:

"You are a white woman."

# `` I want to greet this way!"

I think that some of the notes I made during the months that followed reveal Luke's basic conflicts, as well as the progress he made toward a more realistic version of life.

. . . Luke took off his shoes today for the first time. It was a complicated ceremony. He untied his right shoelace first, then the left. Both laces had to be loosened to a precise degree. With great delicacy, he removed the right shoe, as if he were handling Cinderella's glass slipper. Then the left, in the same way. Before he put them down, he examined each shoe critically and thoroughly—its sole, its heel, its lacing. He then pulled off his socks, wadded them up, and stuffed one into each of the shoes. And then began the placement problem. First, he aligned the shoes side by side with the toes pointing toward the door. Apparently satisfied, he got up from his chair and began an exercise with me. But he kept glancing anxiously back at the shoes, and soon went over to place them with the heels together, toes pointing to the sides à la Chaplin, laces draped artistically over their sides. This procedure went on and on and on, interspersed with outbreaks of his mannerism and only brief and distracted attempts to work. His main concern seemed to be that each of his shoes would look at least once into all four corners of the earth. But at least he took the darn things off. And what's more, he said "Good morning," and made his "horns" bow at me. It was quite a day.

... Luke always enters the room like someone who hasn't the right to come in. He *steals* in, as softly as a cat. But I think that his insecurity is tinged with curiosity. Today, there was the same preoccupation with his shoes. Once more, I asked him to sit down on the floor with me, and for the first time he made it. It was a very complicated maneuver, interrupted countless times by his getting up to rearrange the shoes to every point of the compass, and by frequent performances of his mannerism. But I feel that the ice has been broken. Luke speaks now, although very little. He does take off his shoes. He will sit on the floor. His eyes follow me a bit more closely under their downcast lids.

... Today the shoe-mannerism and the sitting-down procedures were not quite so involved. When Luke was seated on the floor at last, I quickly brought out the beaters. Before taking them, he went through his whole mannerism several times. Then he examined them silently and carefully. He seems to enjoy rhythms, but can't follow the regular beat that Erica (the pianist) gives. He apparently likes to design in the air with his beaters; at least he smiles when he does it. At the end of the session, he held his beaters to his forehead in the "horns" position and bowed several times. I think I'm going to join Luke in his mannerism and see what happens.

... I told the nurses that I intended to enter his movement pattern. They strongly disapproved. He would think I was making fun of him. I might engender a "psychotic episode." He might never work with me again. Why would I jeopardize the contact I'd apparently formed? I went up to see Dr. Keermuschel.

"Go ahead, if you want to. It's an unusual experiment, but certainly worth a try."

When Luke and I were seated opposite each other, and he began his talismanic mannerism, I picked it up the second time around. Carefully and precisely I made the horns, bowed, sliced at my neck, and brushed the top of my head. There was a pause. Luke's eyes were still downcast. He repeated the pattern, and again I followed it. We did it a third time. Luke raised his head. His eyes looked straight into mine. And he smiled. I smiled back.

. . . Luke smiled when he came in this morning. We worked on runs, walks, skips, and turns. There was a slight improvement. Later, I asked him if he would like to dance to the music Erica was playing. He listened to it for a while, then selected two scarves—a pale blue one and a pink one—and fluttered them about for awhile. It seemed to me that the softness of the scarves might be recalling tender feelings, and that his body was reacting to them with staccato movements—like stuttering in motion. He was growing increasingly excited, so I asked him if he wanted to do his "favorite movements." He went through his pattern several times and I again accompanied him. I told him that he could feel free to do them any time he wanted to. He said, "Oh, OH!" in a pleased sort of way. He made farewell horns at me when the session was over.

. . . The same anxious fussing over shoes today, but not quite so many repetitions of the mannerism. As we were getting up from the floor where we'd been working on stretches, my hand accidentally brushed against his arm. At once, his body went into contortions and his face twisted into terrible grimaces of revulsion.

"Oooh, oh! Don't touch me! You'll hurt yourself! Oh, oh, oh . . . be careful! You'll scratch yourself!"

Patients have resisted my touch before, but never to protect *me* from *them!*

. . . Luke balked today, more than he ever has before. He looked and acted confused. He wouldn't respond to my suggestions. At times, it seemed that he would have liked to follow my movements, but couldn't permit himself to do so. His conflict showed in his grimaces, his wiggling around, his cramp-like actions. But he didn't do so many of his basic mannerisms. He replaced them with staccato up-and-down gestures with his extended arms, like a bird that's trying to take off from the ground and can't. When I said goodbye, Luke apologized with the words, "I'm sorry . . . I'm sorry."

. . . When I came on the ward this morning, the nurse said that Luke had told her he was sorry for having been so cranky at the last session. He had said that his little finger had been hurting him. He came into the studio in his usual way: greeted me with his horn movement, did the ceremony with his shoes, smiled, and said "Good morning." He showed me his perfectly good little finger.

"The doctor sawed it off here," he explained, indicating the middle joint. "Then he found a new one and put the new one on at the wrong place. That's why it hurts."

Gradually he forgot about his finger and worked very well: learned the differences between a round back and a straight back, lifted his head more often. Did his mannerism frequently, and smiled when I did it too. Couldn't find the difference between a strong walk and a soft walk. When I asked him to show me how a strong man walks, he said,

"I am a girl. Nobody showed me how to be a man!"
But when I insisted on some strong movements, he began to hit his chest desperately. After a lot of difficulty, I finally got him to direct the blows outward, away from himself. He seemed to enjoy that. When he left the room, he thanked me and said, "Merry Christmas, Merry Christmas, Merry Christmas!"

. . . Today I decided to try touching again. Luke was in a good mood, and smiling a lot. First we touched our own body parts in time to a rhythm. When he touched his head, or shoulder, or knees, he doesn't give the picture of touching portions of himself; he looks as if he's touching strange objects. We worked with the beaters for a while, using them to touch each other's shoulders, elbows, knees. We stood up and did a few jumps and hops. Then I held out my hands to Luke and asked him to take them so we could dance together. He looked at them for quite a while, then looked away, muttering his "Oh, oh"s; then back went his gaze to my hands again. At last, very, very hesitantly, he reached out and touched my fingers—not really holding my hands, but sort of petting them in short, light tappings. He still made faces and twisted his body and peeked at me, but these reactions were less extreme than they had been the first time. We did a few more exercises. When the time was up, Luke made his usual farewell horns. I told him that in Switzerland, people usually greeted each other or said goodbye with a handshake, and I extended my hand. He took it. I gave his hand a firm clasp and released it. He whispered, "Merry Christmas," and departed.

. . . Luke was more defiant today than I have ever known him to be. He looked as if he were questioning everything I did, and everything he did as well. He stared for a long time at Erica, examined the piano, the couch, the chairs, as if challenging their right to be there. He glanced at me furtively from time to time. He stood at the window for a long while, peering out through narrowed eyes. I tried very hard to get his attention. He didn't respond. He was one big "WHY?" He started to gaze at the palms of his hands and make frightful faces. Then suddenly he began his mannerism, only this time he added something new: a highly stylized praying position, arms raised over his head, palms pressed flat together—a really beautiful Gothic attitude of supplication. Then the prayerful hands swept forward and downward, and stopped at the point where they covered his genital area. He hadn't taken off his shoes, and he left without a word.

. . . Luke greeted me with his horns this morning, and took off his shoes. He was far away, but whenever I reminded him he would come back and work a bit. For the first time, I noticed his tendency to "freeze" his movements. He would stop right in the middle of a motion and hold the position for quite a long time. He continues to add the praying and the covering of his genitals to his mannerism. His whole manner is increasingly disturbed. Perhaps I've been going too fast with him. I'd better take it easy for a while.

. . . Luke wasn't in very good shape today. We had hardly begun to work, when he asked:

"Why do people have to *do* something with me all the time? I don't want to dance. What do you want with me, anyway? Why don't you leave me alone?"

He went through his mannerism frequently, and when he left the studio, he made just the horns and the bow, and announced angrily:

"That is *my* way to greet! *I want to greet this way!*"

. . . More and more, Luke includes the new additions to his mannerism: the praying and the covering of his genitals (he constantly pulls his T-shirt down over them). Again, he kept hitting his chest with his fists in that angry, frustrated way. He also smacked his thighs with straight arms and flat hands. But somehow, today, his look was more clear and direct. At times, he seemed quite composed. I managed to pull him out of his negative mood, and he seemed to enjoy this session. He said "Thank you, ma'am!" when he left.

. . . Luke was more closed up today than last time, seemed further away. But he only did his mannerism once! I brought in the big mirror and let him look at himself for the first time. He seemed fascinated with his image at first. Then he looked at himself with a jack-o'-lantern grin. He puffed up his cheeks like a blow-fish and frowned mightily. After a while, however, he seemed to become very agitated, and left the mirror. From that point on, he couldn't bring his head up, couldn't look at me, and began again to make his frustrated blows against himself with his fists. I wasn't able to get him to direct his hitting away from his chest and into space. At the door, Luke mumbled, "Goodbye, ma'am," and bounced his most depressed bounce down the hall.

trying to get him to feel their weight. He seemed to suffer and enjoy it at the same time. It was as if he were experiencing something new, yet vaguely familiar. He liked showing me what to do with the beaters, and used much more imagination in his patterns and rhythms. I followed him in his mannerism again, and this time, almost as if he were joking, he ended with a fancy flourish. I brought him back to his ward after the session, and he laughed a lot when I teased him about his posture. He showed me his hands, especially his nails. I suggested that he should brush them. He liked the idea.

. . . Not much change today. Luke becomes more open with me, often says, ". . . if it is okay with you." The nurse told me that he is now working in the yard, and doing well at it. He seemed pleased when I said that I'd like to come and see his gardening. Luke keeps telling me that he wants a job.

"They call me Negro," he says. "There's nothing wrong with that, is there?"

. . . I went to the yard to see Luke's work. He was proud. He showed me how smooth he'd made the earth, and ran it through his long fingers. When he came for his session in the afternoon I decided to work on space patterns. He walked diagonals, zig-zags, and squares all right, but he couldn't seem to grasp the idea of walking a circle. He always left the closure point open and trailed off uncertainly. I gave him my pad and pencil and asked him to draw a circle. It was exactly like the one he had walked; the line didn't join. As he continued to try, he began to add little designs of his own. Apparently, Luke likes to sketch.

. . . Another commitment caused me to be absent from the hospital for a few days. When I returned, Luke had grown a fancy mustache. He was in a very good mood. He showed me in gestures the work he used to do. It looked like threshing wheat. Then he told me about the little plants he once grew, and I asked him to show me how he did it. The task was involved and involving—beautiful to watch. Luke set his "seedlings" in a straight line from one end of the studio to the other. Two plants had to be placed quite close, diagonally opposite each other. The space between had to be exactly measured. He dug the holes with his hands, picked up each plant carefully, and described it to me as he settled it into the earth.

"This one has bluish-purple flowers . . . this one is pinkish-beige. This one is yellow, with a sort of green in it." The color differences of each plant were described precisely and in loving detail.

Luke spent a whole hour in the fantasy, planting his rainbow-hued garden. Afterward, he said:

"I have a father and a mother. There are three hundred in the family." Then he corrected himself, "Oh, oh-oh, I mean I have two brothers and two sisters. We are five. I lived in a big town in Africa; Kenya, I think it was called. I also lived in Texas. The camps there are very beautiful."

Luke didn't do his mannerism once today!

When he left, he said, "I am very grateful that I met you. You sure are beautiful."


. . . Today Luke's nice mustache was gone. When I asked him about it, he said in a low voice:

"They didn't have time."

He was very depressed—couldn't follow me, couldn't concentrate, kept his head lowered, and wouldn't look up. I asked what was bothering him.

"Why don't I have a dress on?" he replied very sadly. "Why do I have to come here like this?"

I told him that what he was wearing was called a gym suit.

"Oh. Gym suit . . . I would like to be dressed like a man. What am I, anyway, a woman or a man?"

I assured him that he was a man, and asked him to invite me to dance. Suddenly, he was more sure of himself. It was a big change! He took my hand, smiled, and danced me about wildly in a way that Erica told me later was called a jitterbug!

On the way back to his ward, we stopped to see his garden in the yard again. As we stood there, he suddenly became angry.

"I would give my life for the white man. Why are you so nice to me? Why do you mix in with my life? Why do people do things with me? What's the use?" Then he added, "I like you okay."

"I like you too, Luke."

"Goodbye, ma'am."

. . . In the morning, I visited Luke in the yard and showed him some little seedlings I brought for him to plant. He didn't seem too pleased.

"I don't know; I'll have to ask my boss. I can't do anything unless he says so, and he just told me to pull all the plants in the courtyard out."

In the afternoon, Luke seemed worried and depressed. I asked him what he would most like to do today.

"I want to work for the white man."

"How would you begin?" I asked.

"I would greet him," and he made his horns and bowed.

"And then?"

"I would greet him again," Luke replied, crossing his arms over his chest and bowing much deeper.

"And then?" I asked again.

"I would greet him again." This time he bowed clear down to the floor, then straightened up, and said, "That's too much. That's going too far!"

"I think so too, Luke." And we both laughed.

Next, he acted out his wheat-threshing again, and showed me how he dug the earth with his hands, and how he pulled out weeds. All the movements were done with a smooth, practiced grace—a pleasure to see. As he was leaving, I offered him the plants again. He took them, thanking me very much. Carefully holding the box they were in in both hands, he bounced happily down the hall.

. . . Luke talked about a home today: "A home is beautiful."

He thinks that I should have a vacation, and invited me to visit his ward: "It's like a sanitarium."

He wanted to talk to Erica, too: "Good morning. It's a beautiful day!"

He talked almost *constantly* today. When he talks, he can't

Then he began to draw his mother.

"My mother is a schoolteacher. She was a very nice mother. She always wears plain colors. Sundays, she took me and two girls to church. Sundays, I had a dress on. Other days I wore britches."

Luke showed me in movement how he went to church. He bounced and bowed and behaved as if he didn't want to be a disturbance or make any noise—he acted just like Luke. Then he put money in the offering box. He remembered the name of a church song: "Down, Down by the River."

. . . Luke again had a strong reaction. He was very closed in and disturbed today—bent his head far down, froze his movements, didn't want to dance. I had brought him some crayons and drawing pads, but he seemed afraid of them and wouldn't touch them. He did talk about the colors of the crayons, however, making definite distinctions between the different reds, browns, greens. . . . He seemed relieved when I told him that I would put them in the drawer and he could have them whenever he wanted them.

. . . Luke has recovered from the last reaction. He moved well and improvised his own dance very openly, using much more space than usual. The nurse told me that she had let him use the crayons and pad whenever he had asked for them, so I gave them to him to take back to the ward. He seemed delighted, and walked backward down the hall holding them tightly, saying:

"Thank you, thank you, thank you. I sure appreciate it very much. They're beautiful."

. . . "I was in a big society camp," said Luke today. "They used to call me 'white man' or 'king.' It was very nice."

Generally speaking, he worked well, concentrated better than usual. He seemed more pulled-together and serious. But he's so mixed up in differentiating between male and female, boy and girl, dresses and britches! Maybe that's why he says "or-or-or" so much. He just doesn't know what he is. Today, he looked out of the window and said:

"The mountains are very beautiful. You are beautiful, too. I want to settle down, if it is okay with you. You know what I mean . . . ? I can't tell you . . . you know what I mean?"

When he left, I gave him a Milky Way candy bar.

"Thank you and Merry Christmas!" said he.

Luke thinks of the dancing sessions as a job he's been given.

"I am thankful and grateful that I got this job. You know what I mean . . . or, or, or . . . ?"

. . . Another "down" day for Luke.

When I asked him if he'd like to sketch, he said, "I don't know if they want me to sketch."

He smiled when I asked him to dance, but the dance he did was rather fragmented. In departing, he said:

"I want you to be my friend at the very end."

. . . Luke was "up" again today. He had news for me!

"I was a zebra, a lion, a girl before I was a girl and then a boy."

So to close the regular movement session, I asked him to move like a zebra. He just walked around the room. As a lion, he bent his knees more. As a girl, he put his hands on his hips and swayed them snappily from side to side, like a stage vamp. As a boy and a man, his stride was more forceful. He seemed happier, but once said:

"I used to be good-looking. That was before they called me 'Nigger'."

. . . Another depressed day for Luke. I asked him if he had gone to church on Sunday.

"I don't know a church," he answered.

"Did you go to Sunday school, then?"

"I don't go to school any more. And I don't go to church. They didn't want me because I was brown. I don't see why I am here. I didn't want to come here, to the U.S.A. Why don't they give me a job? Nothing is wrong with me!"

"You are here to get well, Luke."

"There is no use in getting well. Now that I'm sick, I never will get well. I don't want to get well. I have no job. Nothing will change."

Luke couldn't move very much; he was terribly cramped. I tried to loosen him up, but he just couldn't relax. I walked with him for a long time. I asked him if he would accept me as a friend.

"If it's okay with you that I am black." And he smiled.

"Regardless of the fact that I am white and you are black, I like you, Luke, and I am your friend."

"I like having you for a friend. But I am worried that you are the friend of somebody else. . . ."

"I have other friends. But I'm happy that you are my friend, too."

Luke wants a home. He wants work. He said he hoped I would get well. He thanked me for everything. It was sad.

. . . Luke had a story for me.

"I met a beautiful woman on the sidewalk. We walked together. She was beautiful. Then I found out that she was my sister."

I asked him to tell me more about the woman.

"She was a beautiful low-class girl."

"How did you meet her?"

"I didn't. She met me."

"How did you find out that she was your sister?"

"I didn't. She said so."

"Did you love her?"

"Yes, I loved her very much. But she said she had a husband, or a boy friend. . . . I want to go home. I want a job. Thank you for the job you got me."

"This isn't really a job, Luke. I'm a therapist."

Later on, he acted out the sidewalk scene. He played all the parts: himself, the low-class girl (beautifully done), and the sister.

. . . Luke had at last been given a haircut; but, as he said, they didn't finish it. The front of his head is almost shaved, and in the back the hair is still very long. We worked on stretches today, and he seemed to be having a good time.

When I asked him to beat a rhythm, he laughed, and said, "I'm not a musician. I don't know how."

But when I joked with him, "Ah, come on now, Luke, you know how, all right!" he made an especially fancy rhythm. Then suddenly, he became disturbed; he began shaking his head and grimacing.

"What's the matter, Luke?" I asked.

"I have a bunch of bees in my head. I don't know how they got in there. I think they came from a foreign country. . . . You are a beautiful schoolteacher. I wish I was a schoolteacher!"

Luke had been sketching maps of the U.S.A. He's very concerned about north, south, east, and west. It's as if he's trying to orient himself. As he was leaving, I gave him a picture book on Arizona, with a lot of landscapes in it. He always thanks me with such touching charm:

"I'm very grateful. . . . It's beautiful. . . . Thank you, thank you. . . . Merry Christmas!"


. . . "I went to school 'til I was five. I was a girl. Then I had a mom and dad. My dad bought me a beautiful suit when I was eighteen or twenty; it had long trousers. When I went to church on Sunday, I had a dress on. I was a girl. Now I am . . . you know . . . sort of a man, or a boy."

"Could you show me, Luke, or act out for me, what you did and how you moved as a girl?"

"I held my left arm with my right hand. And I walked like this!" And he walked about, flouncing up and down.

"Luke, you are a man now. Show me how you walk today."

And Luke walked a masculine walk better than at any time before! Later, I tried communication movements with him. He did very well for a while, but when I asked him to show me in motions that he wanted me to come over to him, he didn't know what to do. He tried, but finally gave up the struggle, and just opened his hands helplessly. Going to the door, he said:

"The boys all looked at the book, and they think you are a beautiful woman. I think so, too. I sure hope you have a good time and get well. Merry Christmas!"

... Luke had seemed to enjoy imitating people and animals, so today I began to pantomime different actions. I asked him to act out pouring some water, then drinking it.

"I get dizzy whenever I drink," he announced. "Even water makes me dizzy. So do all the liquids from trees. I even get dizzy when I eat."

"How do you walk when you're dizzy?"

"I walk just like I walked before!"

He insisted on this quite sternly. Then, after a slight pause, "I'm doing terrific. I mean, I'm doing very good. I'm doing okay. I am sixty now; sixty and forty is one hundred."

"You are forty now, Luke?" I asked.

"I was thirty-nine last year. I never was a baby. I was always alone—I had no father, no mother, no sister, no brother. I was all alone. Wouldn't it be nice to have a family and live in a town . . . you know what I mean?"

We went back to pantomimes. I enacted looking around for something I'd lost, and asked him to guess what I was doing. His interpretation:

"You are looking to see if the janitor did a good job. You are a schoolteacher with a nice floor."

I did another one: I wake up in the morning, stretch, wash my hands, my face, my feet. Luke's interpretation:

"You must have a good time. You met nice people and you greeted them." (!!)

It was Luke's turn. He walked in a circle and made a deep bow. His explanation:

"I paced around on a big stage. It was thrilling."

When I asked him how he would wash his hands, he first plunged his arm downward, as if into deep water, and churned it around.

"I'm looking to see if there are snakes in the water." He washed his hands without rubbing them together. To wash his face, he ducked his head into the water; but he never touched his face. Then he said, as he performed the appropriate actions:

"Now I look up at the sky and see beautiful clouds—very white and hygienic. They come Sunday, then they disappear, then they come again . . . white, blue, pink . . . then they roll

**Black wolf . . .**

184

away." He made soft, rolling gestures as he crawled slowly around—as if he were moving through water. He looked up again and followed the clouds with his eyes:

"They come from the south, but they can't roll back to the south."

. . . Luke had another version of his fascinating past.

"I was a hyena . . . a milkcow . . . a beige dog—the head of a dog family—and now they say I am a human being. When I was a wolf, I met a sheep at the water. It gave me some water to drink. It was a young, beautiful sheep, about twenty-five years old . . . very friendly and nice. The wolf was exactly the same size I am. It was a big wolf."

"What happened then?"

"I made a rag doll. And then I made a grinding machine; and I ground myself . . . and the liquid became grapefruit juice . . . or, or, or . . . orange juice . . . oh, no, it was tomato juice. When you put the rag doll into the juice, it comes alive. Any rag doll you pour juice over comes alive." There was a pause. "I had a sister. I wore dresses. My left leg is my sister's leg. The right leg is my own . . . chocolate and vanilla."

Luke certainly provides fantastic material. I asked him if he would like to act out the same scene with the wolf and the lamb.

"Oh, yes. I want some water. I have to protect my family."

I became the lamb, and Luke the wolf. I scooped up a handful of water and offered it to him. He knelt down in front of me

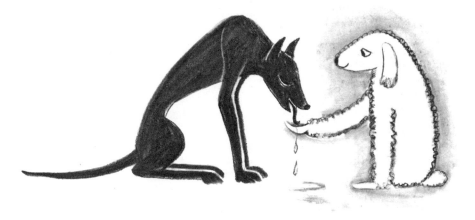

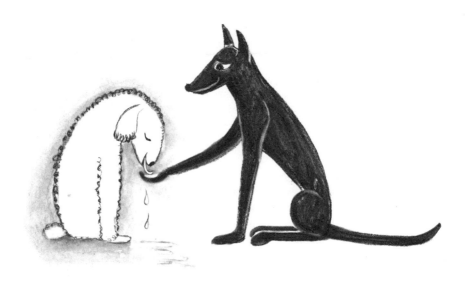

and drank it blissfully. When his thirst was quenched, we jumped
and leapt and ran about like two wolves. His movements and
gestures were marvelous to watch. Finally, we lay flat on the floor
on our stomachs and lapped water from the "lake." Then we
changed parts and repeated the same actions, he as the lamb,
and I as the wolf. After I had drunk from his hand, we hopped
and skipped about like lambs, and again drank together. At last,
we stood up, became erect, and walked together as "ourselves."
And Luke's walk was amazingly different. His step was firm and
secure. His body had straightened out. It was as if he had clearly
grasped the posture difference between an animal and a human.

. . . Luke was very disturbed today. Again, he asked why he had
come, why I had sent for him. He almost refused to get ready
for dancing, but eventually began with the bongo drums, and
started a rhythm. Soon, however, he stopped, and began petting
them. I didn't try to continue. We just walked around the room
together. Finally, he began to talk.

"You are my child. I have many children—as you have.
Where are the children? I know. They are inside us."

He was silent for a while, and then:

"Nothing is wrong with eating people. I like to eat people."

He turned toward me questioningly:

"I don't know who gave birth to me. A woman or a man?"

"Your mother gave birth to you, Luke, and she is a woman."

"Oh . . . my mother."

"You seem upset today, Luke," I said. "Did I do anything to make you angry?"

"You never can make me angry. Never. Not today, not tomorrow. Not ever. I just never get angry with you."

"That's good, Luke."

'That's because I'm a very clever Indian . . . ," he continued. "Oh, oh, oh . . . I think I'm Japanese. What nationality am I?"

"Luke, you are an American Negro."

"I eat people," Luke announced quietly, looking directly into my eyes to see how I felt about this new revelation.

At the end of the session, Luke had calmed down and was smiling again. He wanted me to buy him a pad and some pencils, and insisted on paying for them:

"They don't have your kind of money here."

He thanked me, assured me that I was a wonderful woman, and when he left, said:

"I am now in the eighth grade!"

. . . "First I was beige, then chocolate-brown, and now I am very dark," mused Luke this morning. "I was once a white man. And I think I will be white again. . . . They say this is a hospital. I will be white again."

For the first time, I didn't connect his color fixation with his racial conflict. I felt that he was talking about well (white) and having been ill (dark).

The session began as usual. We worked on levels: exercising on the floor, taking sitting and kneeling positions, and finally standing and moving into space. Throughout the session, Luke was quiet, and more involved in what he was doing. As we parted for the day, he looked at me directly and said:

"I think I'm going to grow up now. It took me six months." We smiled at each other. He started out of the door.

Luke and I had been working together *exactly* six months!

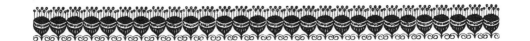

# OVER THE MOUNTAIN
## ``It's Okay to be Dark''

Luke's remarkable time calculation might have been purely accidental. His sensation of "growing up" could have been brought about by his progression through levels in space in our exercises. I'll never know for sure. But within the half year, he had responded so well to our sessions in dance therapy that I thought it was time for him to begin working in one of my groups.

The first two months were marked by regression on Luke's part. Though I had discussed the change with him, he probably felt betrayed. It was obvious that he missed my full attention, and that he didn't want to share me with others. He looked jealous, angry, and finally refused to participate. He didn't greet me any more—no handshake, no horns. He just sat and sat with his dark eyes following my every move. He didn't say my name or call me "ma'am" or even utter, "Oh, ooh." He simply stayed frozen in one position, staring at the session in silence. I was on the verge of giving in and resuming our private sessions, when suddenly Luke made a giant step forward.

One morning, he greeted the room with his horns. A few days later, he definitely addressed his bowing to me. And then one day . . . We were all sitting on the floor. Each one of us had to make up a movement or movement-pattern to show to the others, who were supposed to copy what they saw as exactly as possible. Luke's turn came. Without any hesitation at all, he got up and demonstrated his old mannerism. And I thought he performed those familiar movements with a kind of quiet pride. When the other members of the group tried to do it, he watched their actions like a teacher critically eyeing his pupils' efforts—and he began to correct them. Patiently he taught his wardmates how the movements should be done: the horns accurately and precisely placed on the forehead; the bows performed at a certain angle, deep, but not too deep; the neck gesture executed with sharpness and the head-patting with gentleness. He was master of his "technique," and his pupils seemed eager to learn it. As Luke left the room after the session, he wished me "Merry Christmas."

From that day on, he would move with the group, and again began to talk a bit. He called me by my name. His reactions became more and more appropriate to the situation: he could laugh with the others, and sometimes became annoyed at them. He would skip hand in hand with Sophia, and catch Karl in a race. One day, he brought another black man up to the studio to meet me.

"Trudi, this is my friend, Jack. He would like to dance, too, if it is all right with you, or, or, or?"

There was no doubt that Luke had become an integrated member of the group. He participated consistently for another six months. And although he had his ups and downs, he never regressed to the state he was in when I first met him.

When I knew that I'd be concluding my practice at the hospital in three months' time, I decided to work with Luke privately again. At the end of that period, I jotted down a few final notes. . . .

**I was a zebra . . .
a black wolf . . .**

. . . It seems so long ago that Luke made the remark that gave me hope for his recovery:

190

"First, I was beige, then chocolate-brown, and now I am very dark. They say this is a hospital. . . . I will be white again."

Now Luke *knows* he is in a hospital.

"Everything is very hygienic here. I will be hygienic too—like you are, and like all the people who speak English. Nothing is wrong with me, or, or, or, maybe something *is* wrong with me. But they say this hospital will make me well, if I work hard. I like to work. I want a job."

The road to the tolerance of his blackness certainly has wound through a jungle of confusions:

"You are a white woman."

"Don't touch me! . . . You'll scratch yourself!"

"I am ugly."

"I used to be a good-looking. That was before they called me 'Nigger'."

"I would give my life for the white man."

"They used to call me 'white man' or 'king'."

"They didn't want me because I was brown."

And there were the black-and-white symbols—the zebra, the black wolf with the white lamb.

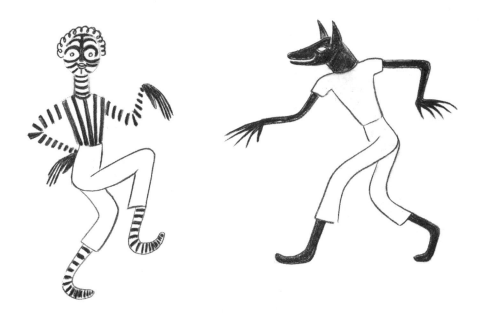

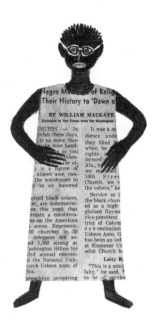

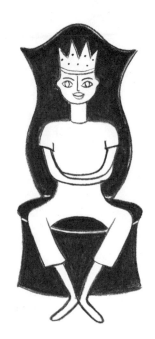

When we started working together again, Luke became completely obsessed by blackness and whiteness. All the other colors of the spectrum, which he had formerly described so lovingly and meticulously, were eliminated from his imagery. He talked of snow and soot, of white eagles and black hawks. He declared he had been a skunk, a domino, a newspaper.

Finally—just ten days ago—Luke abruptly came to terms with the color of his skin.

"My mother is chocolate-brown. My father was an African —very dark. I'm very dark, too. It's okay to be dark."

And that is the last I've heard on the subject! Luke is now aware that he is black and can accept that unalterable fact.

It's been fascinating to watch Luke's physical improvement keeping step with his mental improvement. He now knows all his body parts; he touches them and moves them separately. He knows that he has a front and a back, a right side and a left side. His tension is more flexible, his breathing relaxed, and his posture has undergone a drastic change. He knows that the human being walks upright and that a zebra walks on all fours, and he carries himself as if he's pleased to be human. He can adapt to space conditions, and focus on objects and the people who share them with him. He can express his feelings, both verbally and in movement. Actions no longer prevent him from speaking, and speech no longer interferes with his actions. There is no mannerism anymore. No more bowing to the white man, no more praying to the white God, no more shoe ceremonies. I almost miss all those fantastic Luke-isms!

Luke can distinguish clearly between a man and a woman, and is reasonably sure he himself is a man. When he lapses occasionally into thought distortion, his physical behavior reverts to some of the old familiar patterns, but more and more consistently, he is tightening his grip on reality. His dancing is a pleasure to watch, as he combines the "white man's steps" with his own "black forms and rhythms."

The content of Luke's drawings has also changed dramatically. Those first houses he drew—how lonesome they look, how remote from everything living! When he finally added trees, how stunted and forlorn were those branchless trunks. What excuses he used to give when I would ask him where the people were who lived in his houses: they were asleep, or on vacation, or in the cellar, or in the backyard! How flat those landscapes were, and how sinister the signs, numbers, crosses, and question marks. And the sun, always coupled with the one star: day and night, light and dark, black and white?

When, toward the end of our work together, Luke showed me his picture of the train: himself in the driver's seat, steering his train over the tracks that went high up and over the mountains, I felt sure that Luke himself was on his way over the mountain, and that he would make it to the "other side."

I desperately wished that Luke could have had the benefit of concentrated psychoanalytic treatment; I was sure that I had prepared him for the verbalization of his problems. How unfortunate that this was impossible at the time! However, he had been given other benefits. When I visited the hospital two months later, Luke had been transferred to a progressed ward, where his companions were more reality-oriented. He'd been placed in work-therapy programs, had shown an aptitude for baking, and was now one of the hospital bread-bakers.

Luke greeted me with a handshake, and led me to the hospital bakery to show me the results of his work: eighty loaves of bread, "brown" and "good-looking," were aligned in neat rows, side by side, facing due west. It was clear that he had exercised the same precision with his loaves that he once had applied to his shoes, but this time with a genuine practical purpose, and a lot less time. The loaves managed to look as proud as Luke who stood there beside them, clad in spotless, hygienic white, smiling his broadest smile.

About three months later I returned for another visit, but Luke wasn't there. The nurses gave me glad news. He had been discharged from the hospital two weeks earlier, and was now employed by a baking firm in the city.

Wherever you may be now, Luke, I hope you have a job, a mustache, and a home with a family in it . . . you know what I mean?

Very, very Merry Christmas!

**Luke's drawings**

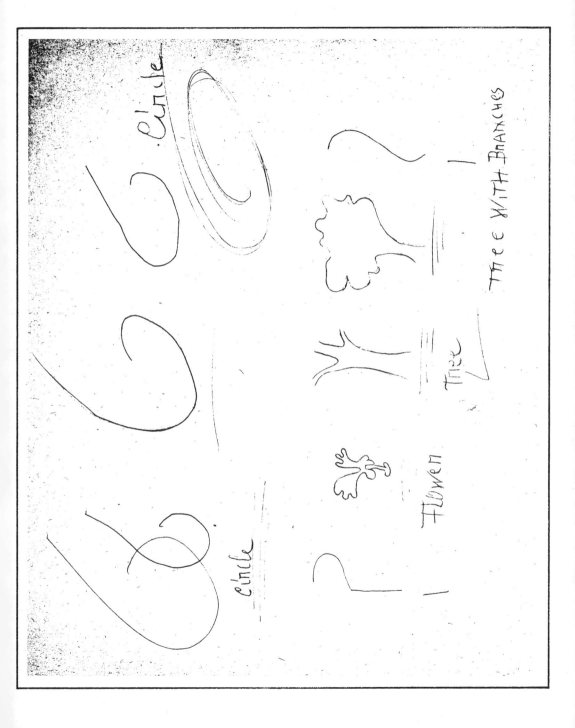

circle

circle

circle

Flower

Tree

Tree with Branches

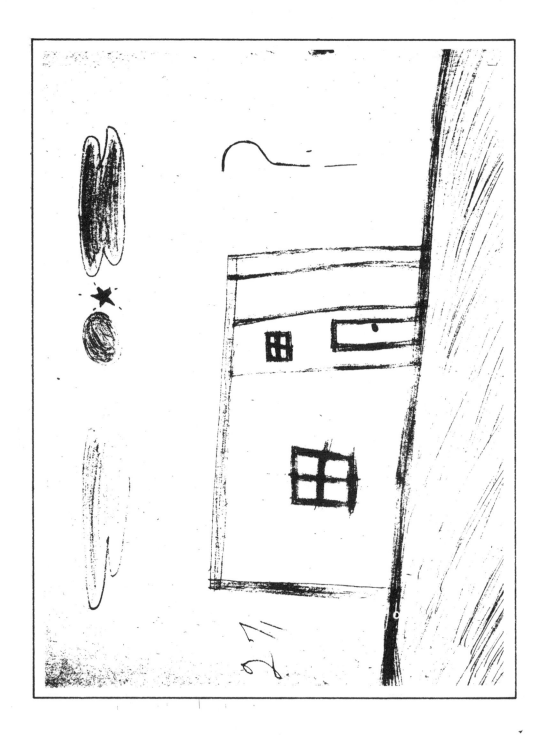

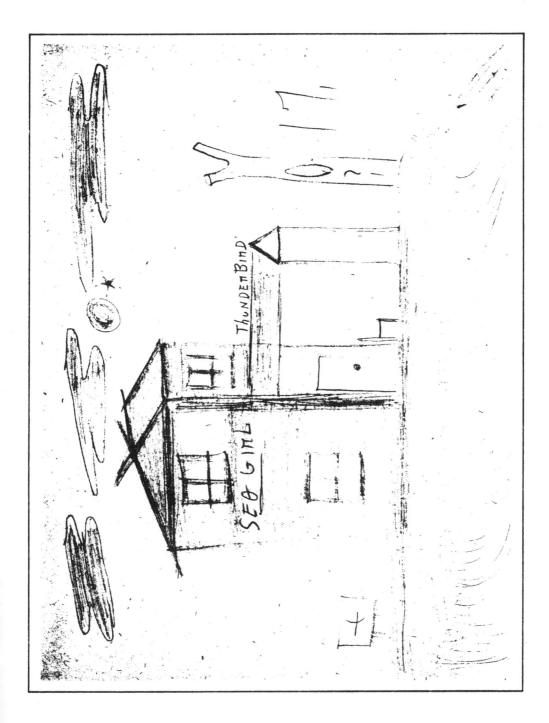

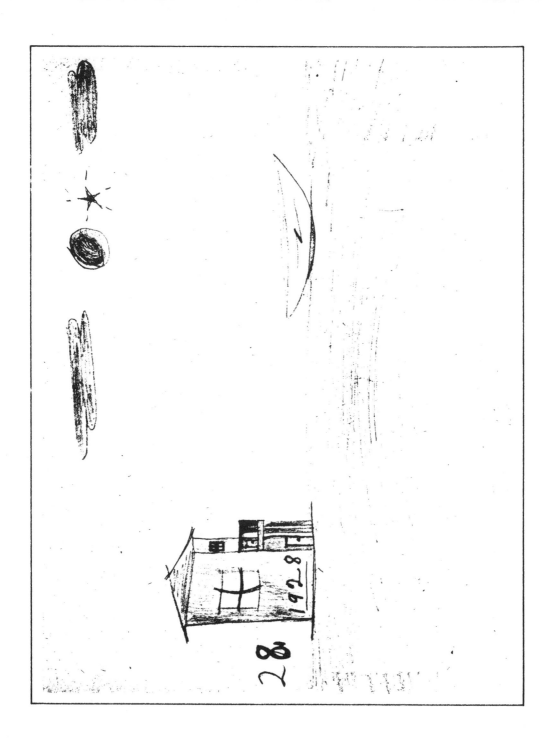

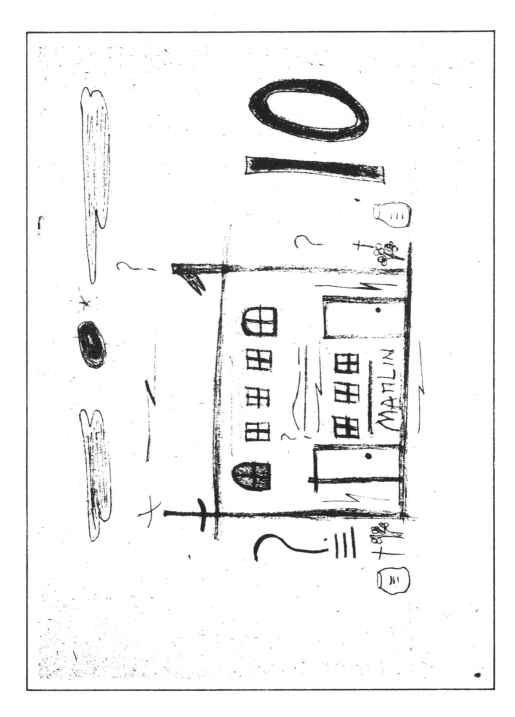

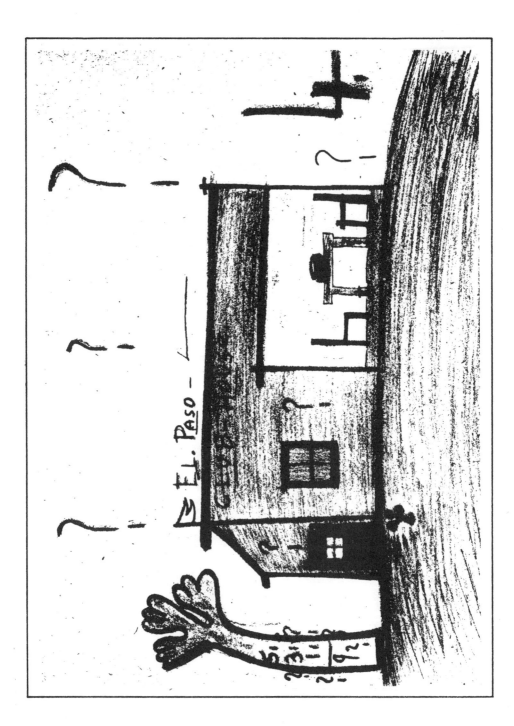

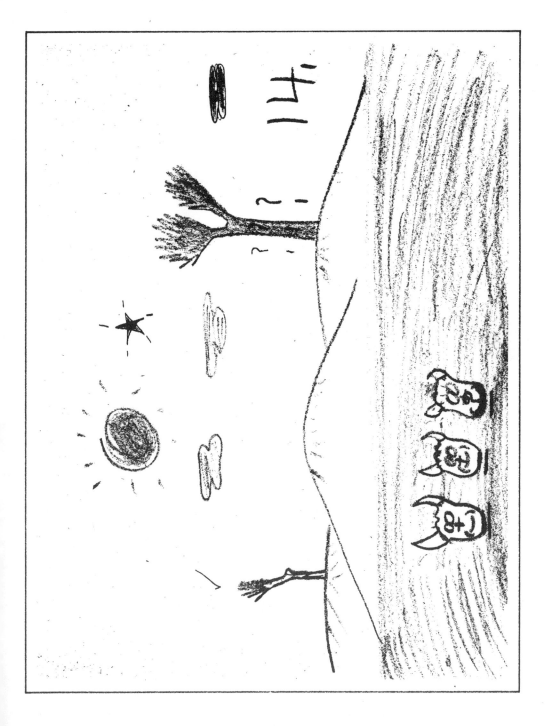

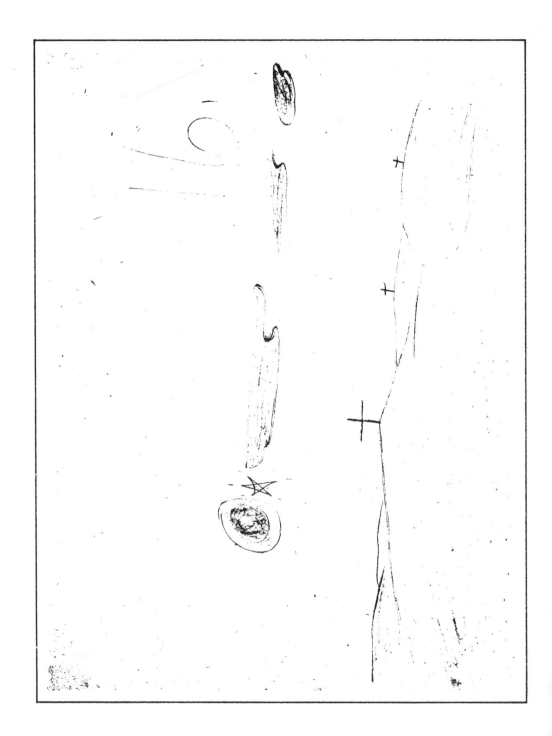

13.

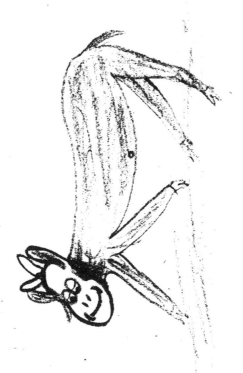

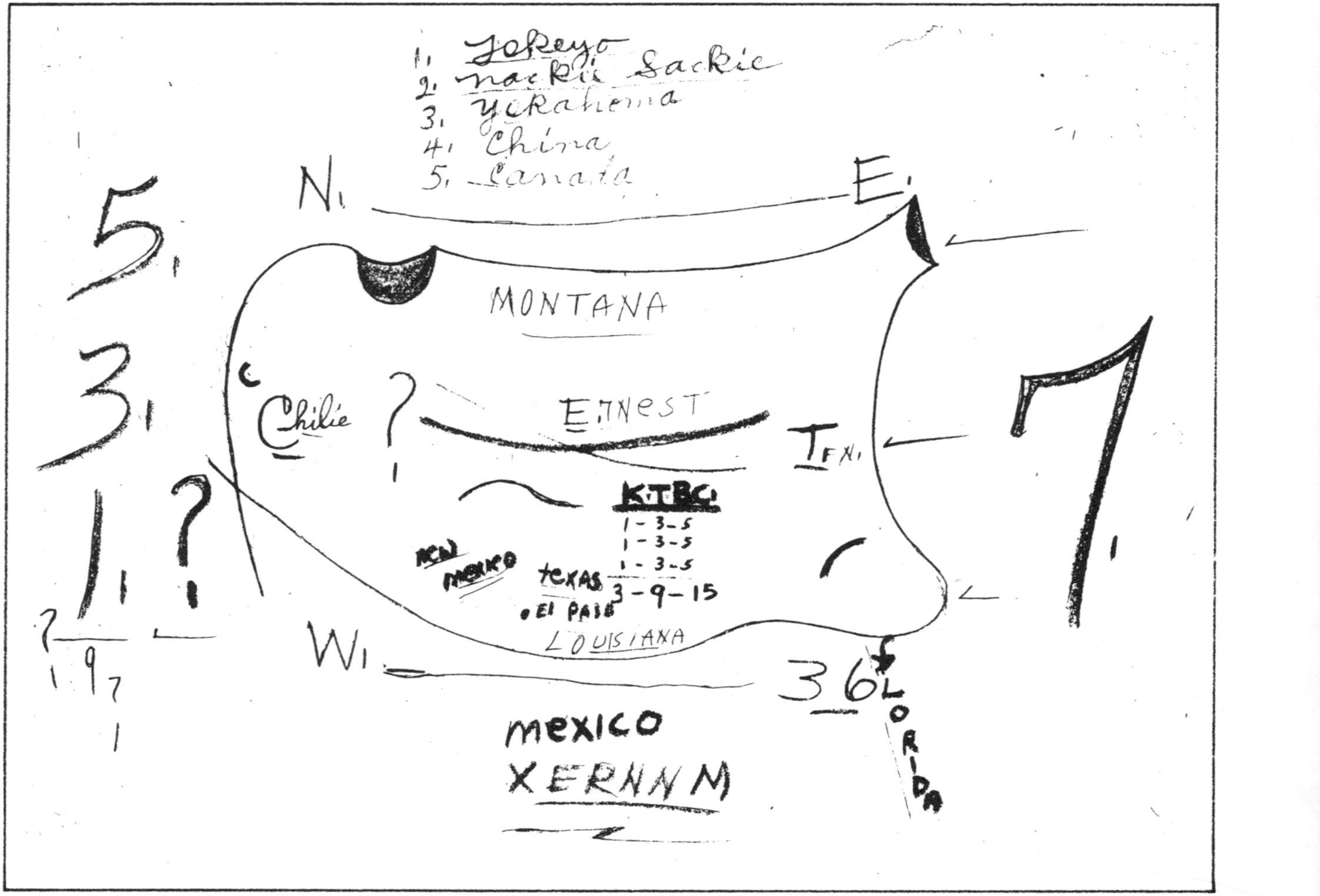
1. Tokeyo
2. nackii Sackie
3. yokahoma
4. China
5. Canata
N.
E.
W.
5.
3.
1.
7.
MONTANA
Chilie
ERNEST
T F X.
KTBC
1-3-5
1-3-5
1-3-5
3-9-15
NEW MEXICO
TEXAS
El Paso
LOUISIANA
36
FLORIDA
MEXICO
XERNNM

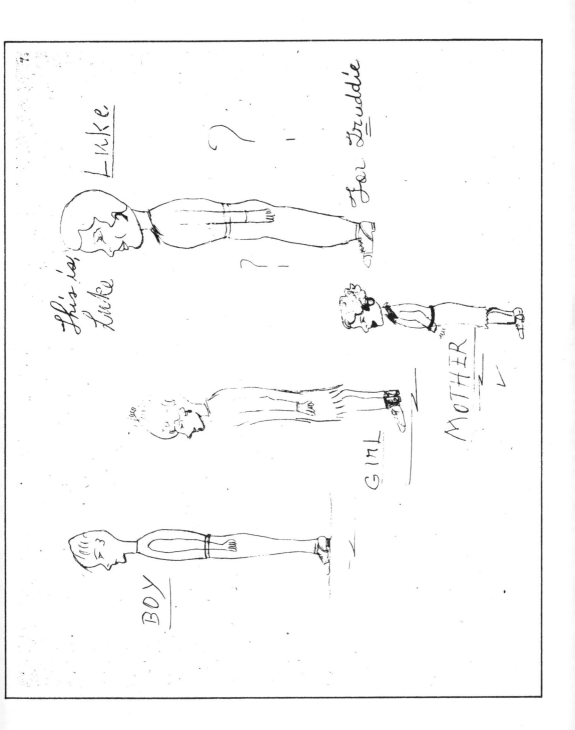

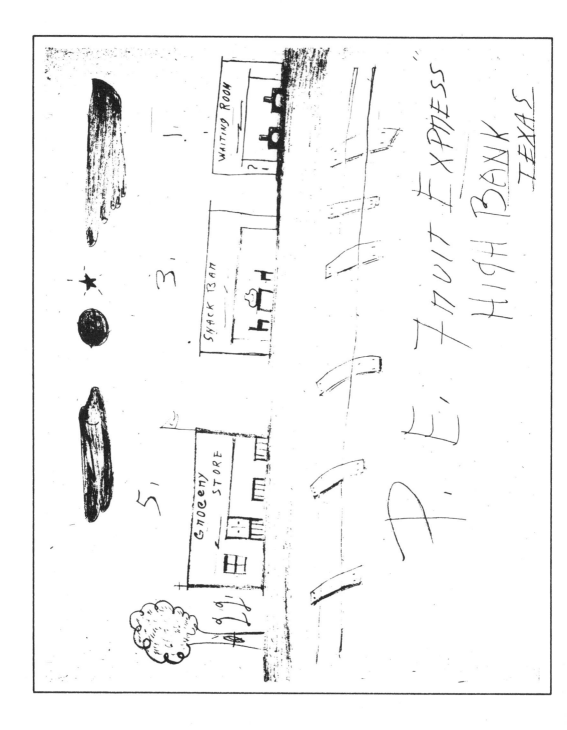

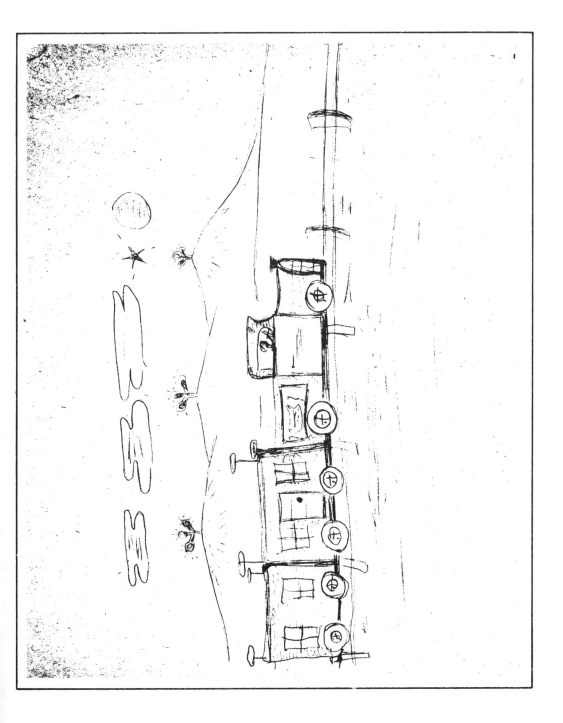

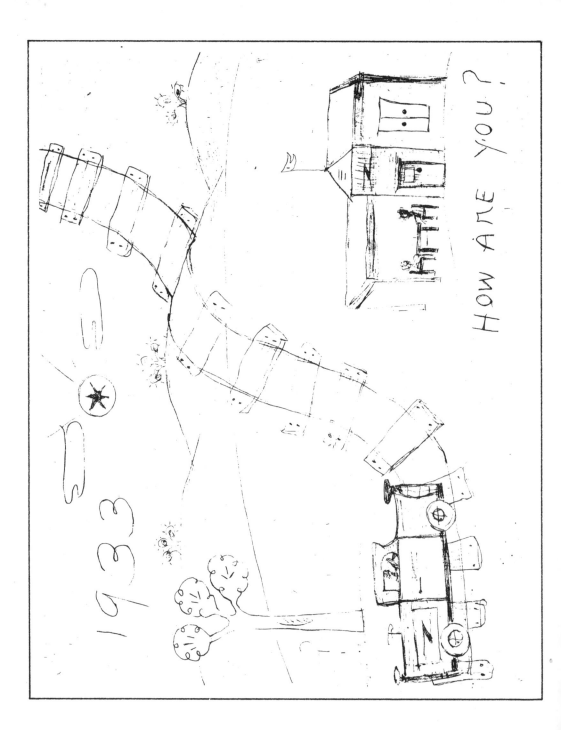

HOW ARE YOU?

1933